Slow Cooker
Delicious & Rapid Weight Loss and a Healthier Lifestyle

(Healthy Slow Cooker Recipes)

Natasha Patch

Published by David Kruse Publishing House

© Natasha Patch

All Rights Reserved

Slow Cooker: Delicious & Rapid Weight
Loss and a Healthier Lifestyle

(Healthy Slow Cooker Recipes)

ISBN   978-1-9992832-4-7

Legal & Disclaimer

The information contained in this book is not designed to replace or take the place of any form of medicine or professional medical advice. The information in this book has been provided for educational and entertainment purposes only.

The information contained in this book has been compiled from sources deemed reliable, and it is accurate to the best of the Author's knowledge; however, the Author cannot guarantee its accuracy and validity and cannot be held liable for any errors or omissions. Changes are periodically made to this book. You must consult your doctor or get professional medical advice before using any of the suggested remedies, techniques, or information in this book.

Upon using the information contained in this book, you agree to hold harmless the Author from and against any damages, costs, and expenses, including any legal fees potentially resulting from the application of any of the information provided by this guide. This disclaimer applies to any damages or injury caused by the use and application, whether directly or indirectly, of any advice or information presented, whether for breach of contract, tort, negligence, personal injury, criminal intent, or under any other cause of action.

You agree to accept all risks of using the information presented inside this book. You need to consult a professional medical practitioner in order to ensure you are both able and healthy enough to participate in this program.

Table of Contents

Part - 1

Introduction

After a long day at work, the last thing any person wants to do is slave away behind a hot stove, swaying on your tired feet. In today's world, we hardly have any time to devote to household activities, the high-powered professional lifestyle cutting into much of our cooking time. Few of us have the energy or the inclination to try making full-course meals!

Slow cookers, on the other hand, allow you to make those delicious dishes as and when you'd like them, while requiring the least amount of attention possible! You could leave your chilly to simmer through the whole day, and when you return from that tough presentation, the food will smell amazing – it's waiting for you to bite into it! Slow cooking has a number of advantages.

For instance, in traditional cooking, a lot of nutrients and natural juices from vegetables and meats are lost – slow cooking requires that you use fresh ingredients that you cook at low temperatures. This means that these nutrients are retained, making your food that much healthier!

They eat up far less energy than conventional electric cookers, they're easily transportable, they're easy to clean up and they keep the food warm even when it is finished cooking by automatically adjusting the settings! For the busy individual who has too much to do or the individual who doesn't like standing behind the hot stove while the eggs are frying in the pan – slow cookers are the way to go!

If you own a slow cooker of your own and are looking for simple recipes to try out – you've come to the right place! In this book, we have listed out for you easy dishes that you can try and make without any hassle.

I hope you find it useful!

Chapter 1: Slow Cooker Breakfast Recipes

Crust less Spinach and Mushroom Quiche:
Ingredients:

- 10 ounces frozen chopped spinach, thawed, drained
- 1 cup Portobello mushrooms, coarsely chopped
- 1/2 tablespoon olive oil
- 2 slices bacon
- 4 eggs
- 1 small red bell pepper, chopped
- 3/4 cup Swiss cheese, shredded
- 1 cup whole milk or half and half
- 1 tablespoon chives, chopped
- 1/4 cup packaged biscuit mix
- Salt to taste
- Pepper powder to taste
- Cooking spray

Method:

1. Place a disposable liner in the slow cooker. Spray the liner with cooking spray.
2. Place the drained spinach over paper towels.
3. Whisk together in a bowl, eggs, chives, salt and pepper.
4. Place a nonstick skillet over medium heat. Add bacon slices and cook until brown and crisp. Remove with a slotted spoon. When cool enough to handle, crumble it and keep it aside. Discard the fat left behind in the skillet.
5. Add oil to the same pan. When oil is heated, add mushrooms and bell pepper. Mix well and cook until tender. Add spinach and cheese. Mix well.
6. Remove from heat. Add the egg mixture to it. Add biscuit mix and fold it into the eggs. Mix well and pour it into the slow cooker. Sprinkle bacon all over.
7. Cover and cook on Low for 4 to 5 hours.
8. Slice into wedges and serve.

Veggie Omelet:

Ingredients:

- 3 eggs
- 1/2 cup broccoli, chopped into small florets
- 1/2 small yellow onion, finely chopped
- 1 small red bell pepper, thinly sliced
- 1/4 cup milk
- 1 clove garlic, minced
- 1/8 teaspoon garlic powder or to taste
- 1/8 teaspoon chili powder
- Salt to taste
- Pepper powder to taste
- Cooking spray

For garnishing:

- A little chopped tomato, onions, cheddar cheese and parsley

Method:

1. Spray the inside of the slow cooker with cooking spray.

2. Whisk together in a bowl, eggs, milk, salt, pepper, garlic powder and chili powder.
3. Add broccoli, peppers, onions and garlic to the slow cooker. Pour the beaten egg mixture over it.
4. Cover and cook on Low for about 5 hours or on High for about 2 hours or until set.
5. When the omelet is almost done, sprinkle cheese. Cover and cook for about 5 minutes.
6. Chop into wedges and serve garnished with onions, tomatoes and parsley.

Loaded Hash Browns:

Ingredients:

- 4 ounces bulk turkey sausage, uncooked
- 4 ounces ground turkey breast, uncooked
- 2 ounces canned mushrooms, sliced, drained
- 1/4 cup onions, chopped
- 1 medium red bell pepper, chopped
- 2 1/2 cups frozen diced hash browns
- 1/2 cup low fat Mexican blend cheese
- 1 medium poblano pepper, seeded, chopped
- 1/2 a 10 ¾ ounce can condensed fiesta nacho cheese soup
- 2 tablespoons water
- Fresh salsa to serve (optional)

Method:

1. Place a nonstick skillet over medium heat. Add ground turkey and onion and

cook until brown. Try to break up the ground turkey as it is getting cooked. Remove with a slotted spoon. When cool enough to handle, crumble it and keep it aside. Discard the fat left behind in the skillet.

2. Line a slow cooker with disposable liner.
3. Transfer the cooked ground turkey to the cooker. Add hash browns, cheese, bell peppers, mushrooms, and poblano pepper. Mix well.
4. Mix together in a bowl, soup and water. Pour this over the hash brown mixture in the cooker. Mix well.
5. Cover and cook on Low for 8 - 9 hours or on High for 4 to 4 1/2 hours.
6. Serve with fresh salsa.

Irish Oatmeal with Fruits:

Ingredients:

- 1 cup Irish steel cut oats
- 2 1/2 cups water
- 2 tablespoons dried cranberries
- 1/2 cup apple juice
- 2 tablespoons golden raisins
- 2 tablespoons maple syrup
- 2 tablespoons dried apricots, snipped
- 1/2 teaspoon ground cinnamon
- 1/4 teaspoon salt

To serve:

- Maple syrup
- 2-3 tablespoons walnuts or pecans, taste
- Milk

Method:

1. Add all the ingredients to the slow cooker.
2. Cover and cook on Low for 6 to 7 hours or on High for 3 to 3 1/2 hours.

3. Serve with maple syrup, walnuts or pecans and milk.

Chapter 2: Slow Cooker Soup Recipes

Black Bean Soup:

Ingredients:

- 1 1/2 cups dried black beans, soaked in water for at least 6-8 hours
- 1 small onion chopped
- 1 small red bell pepper chopped
- 1/2 tablespoon olive oil
- 25 cloves garlic, minced
- Salt to taste
- Pepper powder to taste
- 4 cups water
- 1/4 cup cilantro, chopped

Method:

1. Place a skillet over medium heat. Add olive oil. When oil is heated, add onions and bell pepper. Sauté until the onions are translucent.
2. Add garlic and sauté until fragrant.

3. Add black beans to the cooker along with water. Add the onion mixture, salt, pepper, water and cilantro. Mix well.
4. Cover and cook on Low for 8 hours or on High for 4 hours.
5. Garnish with some fresh cilantro and serve in individual soup bowls.

Dal soup:

Ingredients:

- 2 cups yellow split lentils
- 2 green chilies slit
- 4 cups water
- Salt to taste
- 1 teaspoon oil
- 1 teaspoon turmeric powder
- 1 teaspoon mustard seed
- 1 tablespoon chopped curry leaves
- Coriander leaves to sprinkle

Method:

1. Start by soaking the dal in water for 30 minutes.
2. Meanwhile, add the oil to the slow cooker and once it heats, toss in the mustard and curry leaves.
3. Once it starts to splutter, add in the water, salt, turmeric and chili and mix.
4. Now add in the soaked lentils and mix it around.
5. Add the lid and lower the heat.

6. Cook on the lowest setting for 3 hours.
7. Once done, use a ladle to mash the dal.
8. Sprinkle the coriander leaves on top
    and serve.

Potato and Corn Chowder:

Ingredients:

- 12 ounces red potatoes, diced
- 8 ounce frozen corn
- 3 cups vegetable stock
- 1 1/2 tablespoons all-purpose flour
- 1 tablespoon unsalted butter
- 1/2 teaspoon onion powder
- 1/4 teaspoon garlic powder
- 1/2 teaspoon dried oregano
- 1/2 teaspoon dried thyme
- Salt to taste
- Freshly ground black pepper powder to taste
- 2 tablespoons heavy cream.

Method:

1. Add potatoes, corn and flour the slow cooker. Mix well. Add rest of the ingredients except butter and cream.
2. Cover and cook on Low for 7 -8 hours or on high for 3 - 4 hours.

3. Ladle into individual bowls. Serve hot
   immediately.

Vegetable Minestrone Soup:

Ingredients:

- 1 small onion, diced
- 2 medium carrots, peeled, sliced
- 2 cloves garlic, minced
- 1/2 a 28 ounce can diced tomatoes
- 1 can (15 ounce) cannellini beans, drained, rinsed
- 2 cups vegetable stock
- 2 cups water
- 1/2 cup frozen green peas
- 6 thin asparagus spears, stems removed, cut into thirds
- 4 ounces uncooked ditalini pasta
- 3 ounce fresh spinach
- 3 tablespoons freshly grated Romano cheese + extra for topping
- Salt to taste
- Pepper powder to taste

Method:

1. Add onion, carrots, garlic, tomatoes, beans, stock and water to the slow cooker.
2. Cover and cook on low for 5-6 hours.
3. During the last 15 - 50 minutes of cooking, add asparagus, spinach, peas, salt, pepper and pasta. Taste and adjust the seasoning.
4. Ladle into individual soup bowls. Garnish with cheese and serve immediately.

Moroccan Chicken and Butternut Squash Soup:

Ingredients:

- 2 chicken thighs, skinless, boneless, chopped into bite sized pieces
- 1/2 cup onions, chopped
- 1 1/2 cups butternut squash, peeled, cubed into 1/2 inch pieces
- 1/2 teaspoon ground cumin
- 1/8 teaspoon ground cinnamon
- 1/8 teaspoon red chili flakes
- 1 tablespoons tomato paste, unsalted
- 2 cups chicken stock or fat free low sodium chicken broth
- 3 tablespoons couscous, uncooked
- Salt to taste
- 1 small zucchini, quartered lengthwise, sliced into 3/4 inch pieces
- 1 teaspoon orange zest, grated
- 1/4 cup fresh basil, chopped

Method:

1. Add all the ingredients except zest and basil to the slow cooker. Mix well
2. Cover and cook on Low for 7-8 hours. Add basil and zest (retain a little basil to garnish)
3. Ladle into individual bowls and serve hot garnished with basil.

Chapter 3: Slow Cooker Dump Meals

Recipes

These recipes are called Dump Meals because generally all the ingredients are dumped into the crockpot and then cooked. Alternately all the ingredients are place in a 1 gallon freezer bag and frozen. The bag is then placed in the refrigerator overnight to thaw. Then the ingredients are dumped into the crock-pot and cooked.

Caribbean Dump Chicken:

Ingredients:

- 3/4 pound chicken pieces, skinless
- 4 ounces pineapple chunks in juice
- 1/4 cup orange juice
- 1/4 cup golden raisins
- 2 tablespoons orange juice
- 1/4 teaspoon ground or grated nutmeg

Method:

1. Dump all the ingredients in the slow cooker. Mix well and cover the chicken with the ingredients.
2. Cover and cook on Low for 6 - 8 hours or on High for 4-5 hours or until done.
3. Serve hot.

Hoisin Chicken:

Ingredients:

- 6 chicken thighs, skinless
- 1 tablespoon quick cooking tapioca
- Salt to taste
- Pepper powder to taste
- 8 ounce packaged, frozen broccoli vegetable blend (stir-fried)
- 1/4 cup hoisin sauce or to taste
- 2 tablespoons water
- Cooking spray
- Hot cooked rice to serve

Method:

1. Spray the slow cooker with cooking spray.
2. Dump all the ingredients except the vegetables in the slow cooker. Mix well and cover the chicken with the ingredients.
3. Cover and cook on Low for 6 - 8 hours or on High for 4-5 hours or until done.

Add vegetables during the last 45 minutes of the cooking.

4. Serve hot with hot rice.

Marinara Chicken and Vegetables:

Ingredients:

- 1 pound chicken breasts, skinless, boneless
- 2 tomatoes, chopped
- 1 small zucchini, diced
- 1 small bell pepper, seeded, diced
- 2 cloves garlic, peeled, crushed
- 2 medium ribs celery, diced
- 1/2 an 18 ounce jar low sodium marinara sauce
- 1/2 teaspoon dried basil
- 1/2 teaspoon dried thyme
-

Method:

1. Dump all the ingredients in the slow cooker. Mix well and cover the chicken with the ingredients.
2. Cover and cook on Low for 6 - 8 hours or on High for 4-5 hours or until done.
3. Serve hot

Slow Cooker Salsa Chicken:

Ingredients:

- 1 pound chicken breasts, boneless, skinless
- 1/2 cup salsa homemade or store bought
- 1/2 cup onions, finely chopped
- 1/4 cup carrots, shredded
- 1/2 cup diced, canned, low sodium tomatoes
- 1 tablespoon taco seasoning or to taste
- 2 tablespoons low fat sour cream
- 1/2 cup water

Method:

1. Place the chicken in the slow cooker. Season with taco seasoning. Place the vegetables in layers over the chicken. Finally, layer with salsa.
2. Pour water over the mixture. Cover and cook on Low for 6 - 8 hours or until cooked.

Honey Teriyaki Chicken:

Ingredients:

- 3 chicken breasts
- 1 teaspoon garlic, sliced
- 1/2 cup onions, chopped
- 1 tablespoon olive oil
- 1/4 cup soy sauce
- 1/4 cup ketchup
- 1/4 cup honey
- 1/2 teaspoon cayenne pepper
- 2 teaspoons cornstarch
- 1/4 cup water

Method:

1. Dump all the ingredients except cornstarch and water in the slow cooker. Mix well and cover the chicken with the ingredients.
1. Cover and cook on Low for 6 - 8 hours or on High for 3 - 4 hours or until done. Mix together in a small bowl flour and water. Add this stirring constantly

during the last 15 minutes of the cooking.

Mexican Meatball Stew:

Ingredients:

- 1 can (14 1/2 ounce) Mexican style stew tomatoes, along with its juices.
- 1/2 a c15 ounce can black beans, rinsed, drained
- 1 package (12 ounce) frozen cooked Italian style turkey meatballs, thawed
- 1/2 a 14 ounce can seasoned chicken broth with roasted garlic
- 1/2 a 10 ounce package whole corn kernels, thawed
- 2 tablespoons fresh oregano (optional)

Method:

1. Add all the ingredients to a slow cooker. Mix well.
2. Cover and cook on Low for 6 - 7 hours or on High for 3 - 3 1/2 hours.
3. Garnish with fresh oregano if you are using.

Slow cooked Tilapia:

Ingredients:

- 8 tilapia fillets
- ¼ cup garlic butter, chopped into 8 small cubes
- 2 teaspoons garlic, minced
- 2 teaspoons parsley, minced
- Salt to taste
- Pepper powder to taste

Method:

1. Lay the fillets in the middle of the crock-pot.
2. Season with salt and pepper.
3. Place a cube of butter on each of the fillet. Sprinkle the minced garlic and parsley over the fish.
4. Wrap an aluminum foil all around the fish. Seal it well.
5. Set the crock-pot at Low for 4 hours or High for 2 hours.
6. Serve hot.

Beef Stroganoff:

Ingredients:

- 1 pound frozen stew meat, chopped into bite sized pieces
- 2 cups mushrooms, sliced
- 1/2 a 10 3/4 ounce can cream of mushroom soup
- 1/2 package onion soup mix
- 6 ounces canned ginger ale
- 1 tablespoon corn starch
- 2 tablespoons water
- 4 ounces sour cream at room temperature
- Cooked, hot egg noodles to serve

Method:

1. Dump all the ingredients except sour cream, cornstarch and water in the slow cooker. Mix well and cover the chicken with the ingredients.
2. Cover and cook on Low for 6 - 8 hours or on High for 3 - 4 hours or until done. Mix together in a small bowl flour and

water. Add this stirring constantly during the last 15 minutes of the cooking.

3. Add sour cream and mix well.
4. Serve stroganoff over hot egg noodles.

Country Pork and Mushrooms:

Ingredients:

- 1 pound country style ribs, boneless
- 2 ounces mushrooms, sliced
- 1/2 can cream of mushroom soup
- 1/2 envelope mushroom gravy mix
- 1/4 teaspoon paprika
- Salt to taste
- Pepper powder to taste
- 2 teaspoons flour
- 2 tablespoons water

Method:

2. Dump all the ingredients except flour and water in the slow cooker. Mix well and cover the pork with the ingredients.
3. Cover and cook on Low for 7 - 9 hours or on High for 5 - 6 hours or until done. Mix together in a small bowl flour and water. Add this stirring constantly during the last 15 minutes of the cooking.

4. Serve hot with mashed potatoes.

Cajun Seasoned Vegetarian Gumbo

Ingredients:

- 1 can (15 ounce) black beans, rinsed, drained
- 1/2 a 28 ounce can diced fire roasted tomatoes with its juices
- 1 cup frozen cut okra
- 1/2 a 16 ounce package frozen sweet pepper and onion stir fry vegetables
- 1 1/2 teaspoons Cajun seasoning or to taste
- Snipped chives to garnish
- Hot cooked brown rice to serve

Method:

1. Dump all the ingredients in the slow cooker. Mix well.
2. Cover and cook on Low for 6 - 7hours or on High for 3 - 4 hours or until done.
3. Serve hot with hot brown rice garnished with chives.

Root Vegetable Stew:

Ingredients:

- 1 medium white onion, chopped
- 1/2 pound carrots, peeled, chopped
- 1/2 pound parsnips, peeled, chopped
- 1/2 pound butternut squash, peeled, seeded, chopped
- 1/2 pound Yukon gold potatoes, peeled, chopped
- 1/2 pound sweet potatoes, peeled chopped
- 4 cloves garlic, peeled thinly sliced
- 1 celery rib, stem removed, chopped
- 1 cup kale, remove hard stems and ribs, chopped
- 1 teaspoon fresh sage leaves, chopped
- 2 cups vegetable broth
- 1 bay leaf
- Salt to taste
- Pepper powder to taste
- 2 tablespoons parmesan cheese to serve (optional)

Method:

1. Dump all the ingredients except kale in the slow cooker. Mix well.
2. Cover and cook on Low for 6 - 7hours or on High for 3 - 4 hours or until done. During the last 15 minutes, add kale, mix well, cover and cook until the kale wilts.
3. Serve hot garnished with Parmesan cheese.

Chapter 4: Slow Cooker Meat - Dinner Recipes

Cheesy Spaghetti with Turkey Sausage:
Ingredients:

To make turkey sausage:
- 1 1/2 pounds ground turkey
- 1 1/2 teaspoons dried sage
- 1 1/2 teaspoons dried oregano
- 1/2 teaspoon cayenne pepper
- 1 teaspoon garlic powder
- 1 teaspoon freshly ground black pepper

For cheesy spaghetti:
- 1 1/2 jars (24 ounce each) marinara spaghetti sauce, unsweetened
- 12 ounces whole wheat spaghetti
- 1 1/2 cup low fat ricotta cheese
- 1 1/2 cup mozzarella cheese, shredded
- 1 1/2 cup low cottage cheese

- 1 1/2 tablespoons fresh basil, chopped or 1 1/2 teaspoons dried basil
- 1 1/2 teaspoons dried oregano
- Salt to taste
- Freshly ground black pepper to taste

Method:

1. To make sausage: Add all the ingredients of the sausage to a bowl and mix well.
2. Place a large skillet over medium heat. Add turkey mixture. Cook until it is no more pink, simultaneously breaking the turkey into smaller pieces. Remove from the pan with a slotted spoon and set aside. Discard any fat that is left behind in the pan.
3. Mix turkey with marinara and rest of the ingredients and place in the slow cooker.
4. Cover and cook on Low for 2 hours.
5. Break about 2/3 of the spaghetti into smaller pieces and add to the cooker with the rest of the spaghetti. Add 1 1/4 cups water. Mix well.

6. Cover and cook for an hour more or until the spaghetti is cooked.
7. Sprinkle with more cheese if desired and serve.

Slow cooker Chili Con Carne:

Ingredients:

- 2 pounds lean ground turkey
- 2 medium onion, diced
- 4 cans (15 ounce each) kidney beans, drained
- 4 cans (15 ounce each) fire roasted tomatoes
- 2 cans (4.5 ounce each) green chilies
- 2 cans (6 ounce each) tomato paste
- 4 teaspoons chili powder or to taste
- 1 teaspoon black pepper powder
- 2 teaspoons ground cumin
- Salt to taste
- 1 teaspoon crushed red pepper flakes or to taste
- 2 tablespoons cocoa powder, unsweetened
- 4 cups water or more if required
- 1 cup part skim mozzarella cheese + more for garnishing

Method:

1. Place a large skillet over medium heat. Add turkey and onions. Cook until it is no more pink, simultaneously breaking the turkey into smaller pieces. Remove from the pan with a slotted spoon and set aside. Discard any fat that is left behind in the pan.
2. Add the turkey to the slow cooker. Add rest of the ingredients. Mix well.
3. Cover and cook on Low for 6 to 8 hours or on High for 3 to 4 hours.
4. Garnish with cheese and serve.

Cheesy Enchilada Quinoa:

Ingredients:

- 1/2 pound ground turkey
- 3/4 cup quinoa, uncooked, rinsed
- 1/2 cup frozen corn
- 1/2 a 15 ounce can black beans
- 1/2 a 10 ounce can die tomatoes and green chilies
- 1/4 cup onions
- 1/4 cup yellow or orange bell pepper, chopped
- 1/2 a 19 ounce can enchilada sauce
- 1/2 cup water
- 1/2 teaspoon ground cumin
- 1/2 tablespoon Mexican chili powder
- 3 tablespoons fresh cilantro
- 1 cup Mexican cheese, shredded

To serve (optional)

- Juice of 1/2 a lime
- 1/2 cup sour cream
- 1 green onion, sliced
- 1 jalapeno, sliced

Method:

1. Place a large skillet over medium heat. Add turkey and cook until brown. Remove with a slotted spoon and transfer into a slow cooker. Discard any fat that is remaining in the pan.
2. Add rest of the ingredients except cheese and cilantro. Mix well.
3. Cover and cook on Low for 6 - 7 hours or on high for 3 - 31/2 hours or until the moisture in the cooker is almost dry.
4. Add cheese and cilantro.
5. Serve with lime juice, sour cream, green onion and jalapeno if desired.

Pot Roast:

Ingredients:

- 1 1/2 pounds beef roast
- 1/2 pound carrots, peeled, chopped into bite sized chunks
- 1 pound potatoes, peeled, chopped into bite sized chunks
- 1 medium onion, peeled, chopped into bite sized chunks
- 1 tablespoon olive oil, divided
- 1/2 teaspoon dried tarragon
- 1/2 teaspoon dried thyme
- 1 teaspoon garlic, minced
- 16 ounce beef stock
- 1 1/2 tablespoons cornstarch
- 2 tablespoons water
- Salt to taste
- Pepper powder to taste

Method:

1. Mix together in a bowl, tarragon, thyme salt and pepper.

2. Rub the beef roast with half the olive oil. Sprinkle about 2/3 of the spice mixture all over it.
3. Place a skillet over medium heat. Cook the roast in it until it is browned on all sides.
4. Place the browned roast in a slow cooker.
5. Drizzle the remaining oil over the vegetables. Sprinkle the remaining 1/3 spice mix over it. Transfer the vegetables to the cooker.
6. Pour a little stock to the skillet. Scrape any browned bits from the pan and transfer the stock along with the brown bits into the cooker.
7. Add the remaining stock to the cooker.
8. Cover and cook on Low for about 10 hours or on High for 5 hours or until cooked.
9. Transfer all the vegetables and roast on to a serving platter.
10. Pour the liquid remaining in the cooker into the skillet. Place the skillet over medium heat.

11.   Mix together in a small bowl, cornstarch and water. Pour into the skillet. Stir constantly until the liquid thickens. Simmer for a minute.

Pour the sauce over the roast and vegetables.

Hungarian Beef Goulash:

Ingredients:

- 1 pound beef stew meat, trimmed of fat, cubed
- 1 medium onion, chopped
- 1 small red bell pepper, chopped
- 1 teaspoon caraway seeds
- 1/4 teaspoon salt or to taste
- Freshly ground pepper powder to taste
- 1/2 a 14 ounce can low sodium beef broth
- 1/2 a 14 ounce can diced tomatoes
- 1 teaspoon Worcestershire sauce
- 2 cloves garlic, minced
- 1 bay leaf
- 1/2 tablespoon cornstarch
- 1 tablespoon water
- 1 tablespoon fresh parsley, chopped

Method:

1. Crush the caraway seeds. Mix together in a bowl, caraway seeds, paprika, salt, and pepper.
2. Sprinkle spice mixture all over beef.
3. Place the beef in a slow cooker. Place onions and bell pepper over the beef.
4. Pour broth and Worcestershire sauce to a saucepan. Add garlic and tomatoes. Place the pan over medium heat and simmer for 5 minutes. Pour this mixture over the beef in the cooker. Add bay leaf.
5. Cover and cook on Low for 7 - 8 hours or on High for 4 - 5 hours.
6. Remove and discard the bay leaves.
7. Mix cornstarch and water in a bowl. Pour in the cooker. Stir well and cook on high for about 10 minutes until the sauce thickens.
8. Garnish with parsley and serve.

Cowboy Beef:

Ingredients:

- 1 pound beef chuck roast, boneless, trimmed of fat,
- 1/2 a 11 ounce can whole corn kernels with sweet peppers, drained
- 1/2 a 15 ounce can chili beans in chili gravy.
- 1/2 a 10 ounce can diced tomatoes and green chilies, with its juices
- 1/2 teaspoon canned, chopped chipotle pepper in adobo sauce

Method:

1. Place the chuck roast in the slow cooker.
2. Mix all the ingredients in a small bowl and pour over the roast.
3. Cover and cook on Low for 10 - 12 hours or on high for 5 - 6 hours.
4. Remove the meat and place on your cutting board. Chop into slices and place in a shallow serving dish.

5. Apply the remaining bean mixture all over the meat.
6. Serve immediately.

Middle Eastern Lamb Stew:

Ingredients:

- 3/4 pound lamb stew meat, boneless, chopped into 1 inch chunks
- 1 medium onion, chopped
- 2 cloves garlic, minced
- 3 ounces baby spinach
- 1/2 a 19 ounce can chickpeas, rinsed
- 1/2 a 28 ounce can diced tomatoes
- 1/2 cup low sodium chicken broth
- 2 teaspoons ground coriander
- 1 1/2 teaspoons ground coriander
- 1/4 teaspoon cayenne pepper
- Salt to taste
- Pepper powder to taste
- 1/2 tablespoon olive oil

Method:

1. Place the lamb in a slow cooker.
2. Mix together in a bowl, oil, cumin, coriander, cayenne pepper, salt and pepper. Apply this mixture allover the lamb pieces.

3. Place the onions over it.
4. Meanwhile add tomatoes, garlic and broth to a saucepan. Place the saucepan over medium high heat.
5. Pour over the onions.
6. Cover and cook on Low for about 6 hours or on High for 3 to 3 1/2 hours.
7. Mash about 1/4-cup chickpeas and add to the cooker along with the remaining whole chickpeas. Also add spinach. Mix well.
8. Cover and cook for another 5 -7 minutes until the spinach wilts.

Crock pot Lamb:

Ingredients:

- 2 pounds bone in lamb shoulder, chopped into pieces, separating at the bones
- 2 cups onions, chopped
- 8 cloves garlic, minced
- 4 slices ginger
- 20 ounce coconut milk
- ¼ cup rice vinegar
- Sea salt to taste
- Pepper powder to taste
- 1 teaspoon ground coriander
- 1 teaspoon ground cumin
- 1 teaspoon mustard seeds
- ½ teaspoon turmeric powder
- 2 tablespoon curry powder
- ¼ teaspoon ground cloves
- ¼ teaspoon ground cinnamon
- ¼ teaspoon cayenne pepper
- 2 tablespoons cilantro

Method:

1. Add all the ingredients except the lamb and cilantro to the crock-pot. Mix well.
2. Add the lamb pieces. Mix well. The lamb pieces should be covered with the liquid in the pot.
3. Set the crock-pot on Low for 5 hours or High for 3 hours.
4. When done, the bones should come off easily. Discard the bones and the ginger slices.
5. Serve hot garnished with cilantro.

Slow cooked leg of lamb:

Ingredients:

- 1 ¾ pound leg of lamb, preferably bone out
- 2 tablespoons olive oil
- ¼ cup lemon juice
- 4 cloves garlic, crushed
- ½ teaspoon dried oregano
- ½ teaspoon ground nutmeg
- 1 teaspoon dried mint leaves
- 2 tablespoon white vinegar

Method:

1. Mix together all the ingredients except the lamb, mint, and vinegar in the crock-pot.
2. Coat the leg of lamb with this mixture.
3. Set the crock-pot on High for 6-8 hours until the meat is coming off the bone.
4. With a fork, shred the meat.
5. Sprinkle vinegar over the meat. Garnish with dried mint leaves and serve hot.

Slow cooked Spicy Pulled Pork:

Ingredients:

- 2 pounds pork shoulder roast (boneless or bone in)
- 1 tablespoon chili flakes or to taste
- ½ tablespoon sea salt or to taste
- ½ tablespoon brown sugar (optional)
- 1 teaspoon ground cumin
- ½ teaspoon cayenne pepper
- 1 teaspoon ground coriander
- 1 teaspoon garlic, minced
- ¼ teaspoon ground cinnamon

Method:

1. Mix together in a bowl, the chili flakes, salt, brown sugar, cumin, cayenne pepper, garlic and coriander.
2. Rub this mixture all over the pork roast. Refrigerate overnight to marinate.
3. Place the pork in the slow cooker along with all the juices.

4. Set the crock-pot o Low for 8- 9 hours or until the meat is coming off the bones.
5. Now pull up the meat with a fork and serve hot.

Seafood Gumbo:

Ingredients:

- ¼ pound sliced bacon, diced
- 1 stalk celery, sliced
- 1 medium onion, sliced
- 1 cup green pepper, chopped
- 2 cloves garlic, minced
- 1 cup chicken broth
- ½ a 14 ounce can diced tomatoes
- 1 tablespoon Worcestershire sauce
- 1 teaspoon kosher salt or to taste
- 1 teaspoon dried thyme
- ½ pound large shrimps, cleaned
- ½ pound crabmeat
- 5 ounce frozen okra, sliced lengthwise into ½ inch pieces

Method:

1. Place a skillet over medium heat. Add bacon and cook until the bacon is crisp. When done, transfer to the crock-pot. Discard the fat in the skillet.

2. To the same skillet, add celery, onions, pepper, and garlic. Sauté until the onions are translucent. Transfer to the slow cooker.
3. Add broth, tomatoes along with the liquid, Worcestershire sauce, salt, and thyme.
4. Cover and cook on Low for 4 hours or High for 2 hours.
5. Add shrimps, crabmeat, and okra. Cook for one more hour on Low or 30 minutes on High.
6. Stir well and serve.

Chicken tikka masala:

Ingredients:

- 3 chicken breasts, skinned

- 1 large red onion, chopped
- 4 cloves of garlic, crushed
- 2 tablespoon fresh ginger, crushed
- 1 cup tomato puree
- 2 cups fresh yogurt
- 2 tablespoons vegetable oil
- 2 tablespoons curry powder

- 1 teaspoon turmeric powder
- 1 tablespoon cumin powder
- Chili powder to taste
- Salt to taste
- 1 teaspoon cinnamon powder
- 1 teaspoon pepper powder
- 2 fresh bay leaves
- 1 cup heavy cream
- 3 tablespoons cornstarch
- 1 lemon, juiced and zested
- Cilantro leaves to sprinkle

Method:

1. You have to first marinate your chicken before preparing the dish.
2. Start by adding the yogurt to a bowl along with the curry powder, turmeric powder, cumin powder, pepper, chili powder, cinnamon powder and salt and mix everything until well combined.
3. Now cut the chicken breasts into cubes and add to the yogurt mix. Allow it to rest for an hour or you can also keep it in the fridge overnight.
4. Meanwhile, add the oil to the crock-pot along with the ginger and garlic.

5. Add in the chopped onion and allow everything to sauté.
6. Now toss in the tomato puree and bay leaves and some water.
7. Once that comes to a boil, you can add in the marinated chicken.
8. Add some more water to bring everything together.
9. Now add in the lemon juice and zest and mix well.
10. Close the lid and cook it for 3 hours on the lowest setting.
11. Meanwhile, add the cornstarch to the cream and mix it until a thick paste forms.
12. Now add the paste to the chicken mix and thicken the broth.
13. Cook on low for 5 minutes.
14. Serve with a sprinkling of fresh cilantro leaves on top.

Hearty Jambalaya:

Ingredients:

- 1 can (14 ounce) tomatoes, diced, undrained
- ½ pound fully cooked turkey sausage, cubed
- ¼ pound chicken breasts, boneless, skinned, cut into 1 inch cubes
- 4 ounce canned tomato sauce
- ½ cup onions, diced
- ½ a small red bell pepper diced
- ½ a small green bell pepper, diced
- ½ cup chicken broth
- 1 celery stalk, leaves, chopped
- 1 tablespoon tomato paste
- 1 teaspoon dried oregano
- 1 teaspoon Cajun seasoning
- 1 teaspoon garlic, minced
- 1 bay leaf
- ½ pound medium shrimps, cooked
- 1 teaspoon hot sauce
- Hot cooked rice to serve

Method:

1. Add all the ingredients except the shrimps and rice. Cover and cook on Low for 6 to 7 hours and the chicken is cooked.
2. Add shrimp. Cover and cook again for 15 minutes.
3. Discard bay leaves.
4. Serve hot over hot rice.

Italian Sausages and Peppers with Rotini:

Ingredients:

- 1/2 a 19.5 ounce package Italian turkey sausages, chopped into 1 inch pieces
- 1/2 cup onions, finely chopped
- 2 teaspoon garlic, minced
- 1 medium yellow bell pepper, cut in small cubes
- 1 medium green bell pepper, cut in small cubes
- 1 medium red bell pepper, cut in small cubes
- 1 medium orange bell pepper, cut in small cubes
- 1/2 a 26 ounce jar tomato pasta sauce
- 2 1/4 cups rotini pasta, uncooked
- 3 tablespoons parmesan, shredded

Method:

1. Line a slow cooker with disposable liners.

2. Cook the pasta according to the instructions on the package.
3. Add all the ingredients except pasta and cheese to the cooker.
4. Cover and cook on Low for 6 - 8 hours.
5. Serve pasta on a serving platter. Pour the sausage mixture over the pasta. Garnish with Parmesan cheese and serve.

Chapter 5: Slow Cooker Barbecue Recipes

Applesauce BBQ Chicken:

Ingredients:

- 6 chicken breasts, skinless, boneless
- 1 cup chunky apple sauce
- 1 cup BBQ sauce
- 3/4 teaspoon black pepper powder
- 1 1/2 teaspoons chili powder
- 3 tablespoons brown sugar
- Cooking spray

Method:

1. Spray the pot of the slow cooker with cooking spray.
2. Place the chicken breasts in it.
3. Mix together rest of the ingredients and pour over the chicken.
4. Cover and cook on Low for 6 to 8 hours.
5. Serve hot.

Ginger Beer Barbecue Baby Back Ribs:

Ingredients:

- 2 racks baby back ribs, cut into 2 pieces, rinsed, placed on paper towels
- 4 cups barbecue sauce
- 2 bottles of ginger beer
- Montreal steak seasoning to taste
- 2 oranges, cut into slices along with the peels

Method:

1. Sprinkle top of the ribs with Montreal seasoning and place in the slow cooker. Place the orange slices in the cooker.
2. Pour barbecue sauce and ginger beer.
3. Cover and cook on High for 4 1/2 hours to 5 hours.
4. Remove the meat with a slotted spoon and place on a serving platter.
5. Pour the remaining liquid to a saucepan and place the saucepan over high heat. Boil until it is thickened.
6. Pour the sauce over the ribs and serve

Country Style BBQ Ribs:

Ingredients:

- 1 1/2 pounds boneless pork country style ribs
- 1 medium onion, sliced
- 2 cloves garlic, minced
- 1/4 cup apple sauce
- 2 tablespoons brown sugar
- 3/4 cup barbecue sauce
- Salt to taste
- Pepper powder to taste

Method:

1. Season the pork ribs with salt on pepper on both the sides. Place it in the slow cooker.
2. Add rest of the ingredients. Mix well.
3. Cover and cook on Low for 5 - 6 hours. Remove the ribs from the cooker and place on a serving platter. Discard the liquid remaining in the cooker.
   Top with some more barbecue sauce and serve.

Peachy Barbecue Chicken:

Ingredients:

- 1 1/4 pounds chicken drumsticks
- 1/2 cup barbecue sauce
- 1/4 cup peach preserve
- 1 teaspoon yellow mustard
- Fresh peach, cut into wedges to serve

Method:

1. Place the chicken drumsticks in the slow cooker.
2. Mix together in a bowl, barbecue sauce, peach preserve and mustard. Pour it over the chicken.
3. Cover and cook on Low for 6 to 8 hours or on High for 3 to 4 hours.
4. Remove the drumsticks with a slotted spoon and keep it warm. Pour the remaining liquid in the cooker to a saucepan.
5. Place the saucepan over high heat. Bring to boil. Lower heat and simmer until thickened.

6. Pour the sauce over the chicken.
7. Serve with fresh peach.

BBQ Pulled Pork:

Ingredients:

- 6 pork loin chops
- 1 1/2 cans (15 ounce each) canned tomato sauce, unsweetened
- 1 1/2 tablespoons onion powder
- 1 1/2 tablespoons garlic powder
- 6 tablespoons honey
- 1 1/2 tablespoons apple cider vinegar
- 1 1/2 teaspoon ground cinnamon
- 1 1/2 teaspoon ground cumin
- 1 1/2 teaspoon chili powder
- Salt to taste

Method:

1. Place the chops in the slow cooker.
2. Mix together all the ingredients in a bowl and pour over the chops.
3. Cover and cook on Low for 4 to 6 hours or until it comes apart when pulled.
4. Serve hot.

Chapter 6: Slow Cooker Vegetarian Recipes

Mexican Lasagna:

Ingredients:

- 1 1/2 heads cauliflower, cored, chopped into 1/2 inch florets
- 5 plum tomatoes, chopped
- 1 1/2 cups frozen corn kernels
- 1 1/2 cans (15.5 ounce each) black beans, rinsed, drained
- 1 1/2 jars (16 ounce each) tomatillo salsa
- 1/4 cup cilantro, chopped
- 3 teaspoons chili powder or to taste
- 3 teaspoons ground cumin
- 4 cups low fat Monterey Jack cheese, shredded
- 8 fajita size flour tortillas
- Cooking spray
- Sour cream to serve (optional)

Method:

1. Spray the inside of the slow cooker with cooking spray.
2. Mix together in a bowl, cauliflower, tomatoes, beans, corn, chili powder, cumin and cilantro.
3. Layer as follows: Spread about 1/4 of the cauliflower mixture at the bottom of the slow cooker. Sprinkle 1/4-cup cheese over it. Spread 1/4 of the salsa. Place 2 tortillas over it.
4. Repeat step 3 by layering with the remaining mixture. In all there should be 4 layers.
5. Tear the tortillas of the last layer and place it all over.
6. Cover and cook on Low for about 5 hours or on High for 2 1/2 to 3 hours

Veggie pilaf:

Ingredients:

- 2 tablespoons butter
- 2 cups long-grain rice, basmati rice
- 1/3 cup red onion, chopped finely
- Salt to taste
- Chili powder to taste
- 4 cups vegetable stock
- 1 cup carrots, chopped finely
- 1/2 cup peas
- 1/2 cup green bell pepper, chopped finely
- 1/3 cup almonds, chopped and toasted
- Coriander and mint leaves to sprinkle

Method:

1. Start by soaking the rice in a little water for 15 minutes. Try to use little water so that the rice can fully absorb it.
2. Now add the butter to the crockpot and wait for it to heat.
3. Add in the chopped onions and brown it.

4. Add in the peas, green pepper, carrots and stock and give it a good mix.
5. Now add in the rice, chili and salt and mix until well combined.
6. Now close the lid and cook on low setting for 3 hours.
7. Once done, sprinkle the parsley and mint leaves and serve.

Pinto Bean Stew with Jalapeno Corn Dumplings:

Ingredients:

For the stew:

- 3/4 pound dry pinto beans, soaked in water overnight, drained
- 4 cups water
- 1 onion, chopped
- 1 stalk celery, sliced
- 3/4 cup frozen corn, thawed
- 1small red bell pepper, diced
- 2 cloves garlic, minced
- 1 1/2 tablespoons chili powder
- 1 1/2 teaspoons ground cumin
- Salt to taste
- 1 1/2 tablespoons lime juice

For the dumplings:

- 1/3 cup all-purpose flour
- 1/3 cup whole grain cornmeal
- 1 1/2 tablespoons cold butter, cubed
- 1/4 teaspoon baking powder
- Salt to taste

- 1 fresh jalapeno, finely chopped
- Zest of half a lime
- 1/3 cup buttermilk
- 1/3 cup fresh cilantro, chopped
- 1/3 cup radish, sliced

Method:

1. To make stew: Add soaked beans and rest of the ingredients of the stew to a slow cooker.
2. Cover and cook on Low for 8 hours or on High for 4 hours.
3. During the last hour of cooking, make the dumplings as follows: Mix together the dry ingredients of the dumplings. Add butter and mix until you get a coarse crumbly mixture. Add jalapeno, lime zest and buttermilk. Mix well to form dough.
4. Take about a tablespoon of the dough and make into balls. Drop the balls into the cooker.
5. Cover and cook on High for an hour.
6. Serve in individual bowls with a dumpling in each bowl

7. Garnish with cilantro and serve with
   radish.

Spicy potato curry:

Ingredients:

- 10 to 12 baby potatoes
- 1 teaspoon oil
- 1 red onion, chopped
- 2 cloves garlic, crushed
- 1 tablespoon curry powder
- Chili powder to taste
- Salt to taste
- Parsley leaves to sprinkle

Method:

1. Start by boiling water and poking the potatoes with a fork and adding to the water.
2. Meanwhile, heat the oil in the slow cooker and add the chopped onion and crushed garlic and mix around.
3. Now add in the curry powder, chili powder and salt and 1 cup water.
4. Now add in the potatoes and mix it around.

5. You can add in a little more water if you like.
6. Now cover the lid and cook on the lowest setting for 1 and a half hours.
7. Serve with a sprinkling of the coriander leaves on top.

Mexican Quinoa:

Ingredients:

- 2 cups butternut squash, deseeded, chopped into cubes
- 1/2 cup frozen corn
- 1/2 cup quinoa, uncooked, rinsed
- 1/2 a 14.5 ounce can fire roasted diced tomatoes
- 1/2 a 15.5 ounce can black beans, drained, rinsed
- 1 can (19 ounce) mild red enchilada sauce
- 1/2 cup vegetable broth
- 1/2 teaspoon garlic, minced
- 1/2 a packet taco seasoning
- 2 tablespoons low fat cheddar cheese, shredded + extra for topping
- 2 tablespoons fresh lime juice
- Salt to taste
- Pepper powder to taste
- Sour cream to garnish
- 2 tablespoons cilantro, chopped

- Cooking spray

Method:

1. Spray the slow cooker generously with cooking spray. Place butternut squash in the cooker along with rest of the ingredients except lime juice, sour cream and cilantro. Mix well.
2. Cover and cook on Low for 6 - 7 hours or on High for 3 hours.
3. Add lime juice, sour cream and cilantro. Mix well.
4. Garnish with some shredded cheddar cheese and serve.

Crockpot Lasagna:

Ingredients:

- 1 can (24 ounce) Italian tomato sauce
- 4 thick lasagna noodles with wavy edges
- 1/2 cup red bell pepper, chopped
- 1/2 cup broccoli florets
- 1 cup kale, discard hard stems and ribs, chopped
- 1/2 cup yellow bell pepper, chopped
- 12 ounces part skim ricotta cheese
- 1 cup mozzarella cheese, shredded
- 2 tablespoons parmesan cheese to garnish
- 1 tablespoon fresh parsley, chopped
- Cooking spray

Method:

1. Spray the slow cooker generously with cooking spray.
2. Spread 1/4-cup tomato sauce at the bottom of the cooker.

3. Break the noodles and spread a layer over the sauce. Sprinkle one third of each of the ricotta, vegetables, sauce, cheese and noodles.
4. Repeat step 3 twice more to get 3 layers in all.
5. Spread a thin layer of sauce over the last layer of the lasagna. Sprinkle some cheese too.
6. Cover and cook on Low for 5 - 6 hours or on Low for 3 hours.
7. Once the cook time is over, let the lasagna cool in the cooker for at least an hour.

Cottage cheese in spinach sauce:

Ingredients:

- 1 big bunch fresh spinach leaves
- 200 grams fresh cottage cheese, cubed
- 1 cup tomatoes, chopped
- 1 tablespoon butter
- 1 green chili slit
- Salt to taste
- 1 teaspoon fresh cream

Method:

1. Start by blanching the spinach leaves in hot water.
2. Once done, add it to a liquidizer along with some of the water and the chili.
3. Grind it to a fine paste.
4. Add the butter to the slow cooker and toss in the garlic.
5. Once it browns, add in the chopped tomatoes and mix it around.
6. Now add the cubed cottage cheese and the ground spinach along with some water and salt and mix well.

7. Close the slow cooker and cook on the lowest setting for an hour and a half.
8. Serve with a swirl of fresh cream on top.

Broccoli and Rice Casserole:

Ingredients:

- 3/4 cup brown rice, uncooked
- 1 1/4 cup water
- 1/4 cup mushrooms, finely chopped
- 1/2 pound broccoli florets, finely chopped
- 1 tablespoon butter
- 2 tablespoons onions, finely chopped
- 1 clove garlic, minced
- 1 cup milk
- 1 tablespoon flour
- 1/4 cup walnuts, chopped (optional)
- 1/2 cup low fat cheddar cheese, divided
- 2 tablespoons parmesan cheese, grated
- Salt to taste
- Pepper powder to taste

Method:

1. Place a skillet over medium heat. Add butter. When butter melts, add onions,

garlic and mushrooms. Sauté until the onions are translucent.

2. Add salt, pepper and flour. Sauté until brown.

3. Gently pour milk. Stir constantly and bring to a boil. Simmer for a minute and remove from heat.

4. Add cheese and mix well.

5. Place rice in the cooker. Add water, broccoli, and cheese sauce. Mix.

6. Cover and cook on Low for 6 - 7 hours or until the rice is tender.

7. Uncover, sprinkle both cheddar cheese and Parmesan.

8. Cover and cook for one hour on Low.

9. Garnish with walnuts and serve.

Barley and Chickpea Risotto:

Ingredients:

- 6 carrots, peeled, chopped
- 6 cloves garlic, minced
- 1 small yellow onion, minced
- 1 head cauliflower, cut into small florets
- 3 tablespoons extra virgin olive oil
- 2 1/2 cups pearl barley, rinsed
- 8 sprigs, fresh thyme
- 2 cans (15.5 ounce each) garbanzo beans, rinsed, drained
- 2 1/2 cups water
- 5 cups low sodium vegetable broth
- Salt to taste
- Pepper powder to taste
- 3 tablespoons lemon juice
- 6 tablespoons fresh parsley, chopped
- 2/3 cup parmesan cheese, grated

Method:

1. Place a skillet over medium high heat. Add oil. When oil is heated, add onions,

garlic, cauliflower and carrots. Sauté until the onions are translucent.

2. Add barley and thyme and stir frequently for about 2 minutes.

3. Remove from heat and transfer into the slow cooker.

4. Add garbanzo beans, broth, water, salt and pepper. Mix well.

5. Cover and cook on Low for 5 - 6 hours or 2 - 2 1/2 hours or until the barley is tender and almost all the liquid is absorbed.

6. Discard the thyme sprigs. Add lemon juice.

7. Serve in individual bowls garnished with cheese and parsley.

Chapter 7: Cooking for 2 in a Slow Cooker

Breakfast Recipes:

Overnight Cinnamon Apple Oatmeal:
Ingredients:

- 1 large Granny Smith or Pink lady apple, cored, chopped
- 1/2 cup whole grain oats
- 3/4 cup skim milk
- 3/4 cup water
- 1 1/2 tablespoons packed dark brown sugar
- 1/2 tablespoon ground cinnamon
- 1 tablespoon ground flaxseed
- 1 tablespoon butter
- 1/8 teaspoon kosher salt
- Cooking spray
- 2 tablespoons nuts of your choice, chopped to serve
- 2 tablespoons dried fruits of your choice like raisins etc. to serve

Method:

1. Spray the inside of the slow cooker with cooking spray.
2. Add all the ingredients except salt to the slow cooker. Mix well.
3. Cover and cook on Low for 6 to 7 hours.
4. Add salt just before serving. Garnish with chopped nuts and dried fruits and serve.

Spinach and Mozzarella Frittata:

Ingredients:

- 2 eggs
- 2 egg whites
- 1/2 tablespoon extra-virgin olive oil
- 3 tablespoons onions, chopped
- 1 tablespoon 1 % milk
- 1/2 cup low fat mozzarella cheese, shredded, divided
- A pinch black pepper powder or to taste
- A pinch white pepper powder or to taste
- A large pinch salt or to taste
- 1/2 cup baby spinach leaves, chopped
- 1 small Roma tomato, diced
- Cooking spray

Method:

1. Spray the inside of the cooker with cooking spray.
2. Place a skillet over medium heat. Add oil. When oil is heated, add onions and

garlic and sauté until the onions are translucent.

3. Transfer the onions and garlic into the pot of the slow cooker. Add rest of the ingredients retaining about 1/2 the cheese. Whisk well.
4. Sprinkle the remaining cheese over it.
5. Cook on Low for 1 to 1 1/2 hours or until done.
6. Chop into wedges and serve.

Bacon, Egg & Hash Brown Casserole:

Ingredients:

- 5 ounce frozen shredded hash browns
- 2 slices thick cut bacon, cooked, chopped
- 3 eggs
- 2 green onions, thinly sliced
- 2 ounces cheddar cheese, shredded
- 2 tablespoons milk
- Salt to taste
- Pepper powder to taste
- Cooking spray

Method:

1. Spray the slow cooker with cooking spray.
2. Spread half the hash browns at the bottom of the cooker. Layer with half the bacon followed by half the cheese and green onions.
3. Repeat step 2 with the remaining half of the hash browns, cheese and green onions.

4. Whisk together in a bowl, eggs, milk, salt and pepper. Pour over the layers in the cooker.
5. Cover and cook on Low for about 4 hours or on high for about 2 hours or until the eggs are set.
6. Serve immediately preferably with some hot sauce.

Dinner Recipes:

Shrimp and Artichoke Barley Risotto:

Ingredients:

- 1/2 cup pearl barley
- 1 1/2 cups water for lobster base
- 1 1/2 teaspoons Better than Bouillon lobster base
- 1/2 cup onions, chopped
- 2 cloves garlic, minced
- 1/2 a 9 ounce package frozen artichoke hearts, thawed, quartered
- 1/2 pound shrimp, peeled, deveined
- 2 ounce baby spinach
- Salt to taste
- Pepper powder to taste
- 1 teaspoon lemon zest

Method:

1. Pour water in a small saucepan. Remove from heat. Add lobster base. Whisk well and set it aside. You can

also use 1 1/2 cups seafood broth or chicken broth instead.

2. Place a nonstick skillet over medium low heat. Add onions and sauté until the onions are translucent. Add garlic and sauté for a minute or until the garlic is fragrant.
3. Transfer into the slow cooker. Add lobster mixed with water. Artichoke hearts, pepper powder and barley.
4. Cover and cook on Low for 6 - 7 hours or on High for 3 hours or until the liquid in the cooker has dried up.
5. Add shrimp and cheese. Cover and cook on High for 10 minutes or until the shrimp have turned opaque.
6. Add lemon zest and baby spinach. Gently fold. Add salt and pepper.
7. Serve in individual serving bowls immediately.

Crockpot Quinoa:

Ingredients:

- 1/2 cup quinoa, rinsed, uncooked
- 1/3 cup low sodium canned chickpeas, drained, rinsed
- 1/4 cup canned black beans, drained, rinsed
- 1/2 cup frozen corn
- 1 small red pepper, chopped
- 1 small onion, chopped
- 1 Roma tomato, chopped
- 1/2 tablespoon garlic, minced
- 1 cup low sodium vegetable broth
- 1 teaspoon ground cumin
- Salt to taste
- Pepper powder to taste
- 1 tablespoon sauce from a can of chipotle peppers in adobo sauce
- 2 tablespoons fresh cilantro, chopped
- 2 tablespoons cheddar cheese, shredded
- Cooking spray

Method:

1. Spray the slow cooker generously with cooking spray. Add all the ingredients except salt, pepper, cheese and cilantro.
2. Mix well. Cover and cook on High for 3 - 4 hours. Uncover and check after 3 hours if the quinoa is done.
3. Add salt and pepper. Fluff with a fork.
4. Garnish with cheese and cilantro. Serve hot.

Vegetable Curry:

Ingredients:

- 2 medium carrots, peeled, sliced
- 1 medium potato, cut into 1/2 inch cubes
- 4 ounces fresh green beans, stringed, chopped into 1 inch pieces
- 2 cloves garlic, minced
- 1/2 cup onions, chopped
- 1 tablespoon quick cooking tapioca
- 1/2 a 14 ounce cans vegetable broth or you can use homemade broth too.
- 1/2 a 14.5-ounce can diced tomatoes, with its liquid.
- 1/2 a 15 ounce can garbanzo beans, drained, rinsed
- 1 teaspoon curry powder
- 1/2 teaspoon ground coriander
- 1/4 teaspoon crushed red pepper or to taste
- A large pinch ground cinnamon
- 1/4 teaspoon salt or to taste

- Hot cooked rice to serve

Method:

1. Add all the ingredients except tomatoes to the slow cooker. Mix well.
2. Cover and cook on Low for 6 - 7 hours or on high to 3 1/2 - 4 1/2 hours.
3. Add tomatoes with its juices. Mix well.
4. Cover and set it aside for at least 5 minutes.
5. Place hot cooked rice on a serving platter. Pour the curry over the rice and serve.

Cauliflower Garlic Mashed Potatoes:

Ingredients:

- 1/2 a head cauliflower, chopped into florets
- 1 1/4 cups water
- 1/2 tablespoon butter
- 1 bay leaf
- Salt to taste
- Pepper powder to taste
- 4 cloves garlic, peeled
- 2 tablespoons milk
- Chives or green onions to serve

Method:

1. Place cauliflower, garlic, salt and bay leaf in the slow cooker. Pour water. Mix well.
2. Cover and cook on Low for 4 to 6 hours or on High for 2 hours.
3. Discard the bay leaf. Drain the excess water that is present in the cooker.

4. Add butter and mix well. Mash the contents with a potato masher adding about a tablespoon of milk.
5. Add the remaining tablespoon of milk if required. Season with salt and pepper.
6. Serve hot with chives.

Russian Apricot Chicken:

Ingredients:

- 1 pound chicken breasts, boneless, skinless
- 1 small onion, chopped
- 1/2 a 12 ounce jar apricot preserves
- 1/2 a bottle of Russian salad dressing or to taste

Method:

1. Mix together in a bowl, onions, half the apricot preserves and half the salad dressing.
2. Add chicken pieces to the slow cooker. Pour the apricot preserve mixture over it.
3. Cover and cook on Low for 7 - 8 hours
4. Serve with rice or mashed potatoes. Pour the remaining apricot preserves and dressing over the chicken and serve.

Lemon Garlic Chicken:

Ingredients:

- 2 chicken breasts
- 2 tablespoons olive oil
- 1/2 tablespoons parsley flakes
- 1 tablespoon lemon juice
- Salt to taste
- Pepper powder to taste

Method:

1. Add all the ingredients to the slow cooker.
2. Cover and cook on Low for 7 - 8 hours.
3. Serve hot.

Ranch Chicken:

Ingredients:

- 2 chicken breasts, boneless
- 3/4 cup chicken broth
- 1 tablespoon dry taco mix
- 1 tablespoon dry ranch dressing mix

Method:

1. Add all the ingredients to the slow cooker. Mix well and spoon some of the mixture over the chicken.
2. Cover and cook on Low for 7 - 8 hours.
3. Remove the chicken with a slotted spoon. Place on your cutting board. Shred the chicken with 2 forks.
4. Add the chicken back to the cooker. Cover and cook for another 30 minutes.
5. Serve hot.

Dessert:

Slow cooked Poached Pears in Caramel Sauce:

Ingredients:

- 2 firm Bartlett or Bosc pears, slightly under ripe, peeled, halved lengthwise, cored
- 3/4 cup brown sugar
- 1/2 tablespoon fresh ginger, grated
- 1/8 teaspoon ground cinnamon
- 1 tablespoon butter, unsalted, cubed

Method:

1. Add sugar, ginger and butter to the slow cooker. Add pears and toss. Place the pears such that the cut side is on the bottom of the cooker.
2. Cover and cook on High for 2 hours. Half way through the cooking, uncover and pour the sauce on the top of the pears. Do not overcook.

3. Remove the pears with a slotted spoon and place 2 halves in each bowl.
4. Pour the sauce into a small saucepan. Place the saucepan over medium heat and bring to a boil. Lower heat; simmer for a couple of minutes until the sauce is slightly thickened.
5. Pour the sauce over the pears. Sprinkle cinnamon and serve warm.

Chapter 8: Slow Cooker Desserts Recipes

Rice Pudding:

Ingredients:

- 1 1/2 cups short grain rice
- 2 cans (3 1/2 ounce each) evaporated milk
- 4 cups water
- 2 teaspoons vanilla extract
- 1/2 cup sugar or to taste
- 3/4 cup raisins
- 2 sticks cinnamon

Method:

1. Add all the ingredients to the slow cooker.
2. Cover and cook on Low for 7 8 hours. Stir in between a couple of times.
3. Serve hot.

Sago pearls in sweet milk:

Ingredients:

- 1 cup sago pearls
- 2 cups skimmed milk
- ½ cup brown sugar
- 2 pods cardamom, crushed
- 1 teaspoon clarified butter or ghee
- 2 tablespoons mixed dry fruits, chopped

Method:

1. Start by soaking the sago pearls in enough water for 30 minutes.
2. Meanwhile, add the ghee to the crockpot and once it heats, add in the dry fruits and crushed cardamom pods.
3. When it browns, add in the milk and stir.
4. Add in the sugar and allow it to mix in well.
5. Now add the sago pearls to it and close the lid.
6. Cook it on low for 2 hours.
7. Your yummy sago pearls is now ready to serve. You can serve it as is or chill and serve.

Peach Cobbler:

Ingredients:

- 3 ounce dark brown sugar
- 1 ¾ cup rolled oats
- 2 ounce all-purpose flour
- ¼ teaspoon baking powder
- ¼ teaspoon freshly ground all spice
- ¼ teaspoon freshly ground nutmeg
- A pinch kosher salt
- 2 tablespoons unsalted butter, at room temperature
- 10 ounce frozen peach slices
- Cooking spray

Method:

1. Mix together sugar, flour, oats, baking powder, nutmeg, allspice, and kosher salt in a bowl. Add butter and mix into a crumbly mixture.
2. Add the peach and fold.
3. Spray the bottom of the slow cooker. Transfer the tie peach mixture into the cooker. Cover.

4. Set the cooker on Low for 3-3 ½ hours.
5. Serve hot immediately.

Cranberry Stuffed Apples:

Ingredients:

- 3 medium apples
- 1/4 cup fresh or frozen cranberries, thawed, chopped
- 3 tablespoons packed brown sugar
- 1/4 teaspoon ground cinnamon
- A large pinch ground nutmeg
- Whipped cream or vanilla ice cream to serve (optional)

Method:

1. Leave the bottoms of the apple intact and core rest of the apple. Peel only the top part of the apple.
2. Mix together cranberries, brown sugar, walnuts, cinnamon and nutmeg. Fill this into the apples.
3. Place the apples in a slow cooker and cook on Low for about 4 hours. Do not overcook.
4. Serve with whipped cream or ice cream.

Pumpkin –Pomegranate Cheesecake:

Ingredients:

- 6 ounce low fat cream cheese, softened
- ¼ cup granulated sugar
- ½ tablespoon all-purpose flour
- ½ teaspoon pumpkin pie spice (optional)
- ¼ teaspoon vanilla
- 1/3 cup canned pumpkin
- 2 small eggs, lightly beaten
- ½ teaspoon orange peel, grated
- ½ cup warm water
- ¼ cup pomegranate juice
- ½ tablespoon brown sugar
- ¾ teaspoon corn starch
- ¼ cup pomegranate seeds
- Cooking spray

Method:

1. Spray a soufflé dish (size should be smaller than the cooker) with cooking spray. Line with parchment paper. Take an 18x12 inch heavy foil, cut into 2

halves. Fold each piece lengthwise to 3 folds. Place it crisscross and place the soufflé dish on top of it.

2. Place cream cheese in a bowl. Beat with an electric stick blender at high speed for about 30 seconds. Add granulated sugar, pumpkin spice, flour, and vanilla. Beat on medium speed until well mixed.

3. Add pumpkin and beat until smooth. Add eggs one by one on low speed until well combined. Add orange peel and stir well.

4. Pour this mixture into the soufflé dish. Cover with foil.

5. Pour water into the slow cooker. Use the ends of the foil strips and gently lift the dish and place in the cooker. Cover.

6. Set the cooker on High for 2 ½ hours or until the center is set.

7. Gently remove the soufflé dish with the help of the foil strips. Discard the strips.

8. Cool on a wire rack. Chill in the refrigerator for a minimum of 4 hours.

9. To make the sauce: place a saucepan over medium heat. Add pomegranate

juice, brown sugar, and cornstarch. Stir constantly until the sauce is thickened. Transfer to a bowl. Cover and cool to room temperature.

10. To serve: Loosen the sides of the cheesecake with a knife. Place a plate over the dish and invert the cheesecake on to the plate. Remove the parchment paper and discard.

11. Cut the cheesecake into wedges and serve with sauce over the wedge. Garnish with pomegranate seeds.

Apple Crumble Pudding:

Ingredients:

For the pudding

- 2 cups almond milk or coconut milk
- 4 cups water
- ¼ cup raw honey (optional)
- 1 cup chia seeds
- 4 tablespoons arrowroot powder
- 2 teaspoons ground cinnamon
- A large pinch Himalayan pink salt
- 10 large apples, cored, sliced

For the topping:

- 1 cup blanched almond flour
- ½ cup shredded coconut, unsweetened
- ½ cup coconut sugar
- 2 teaspoons cinnamon
- ½ cup unsweetened apple sauce
- 2 teaspoons vanilla extract

For garnishing:

- 2 tablespoons raisins
- 2 tablespoons walnuts, chopped

Method:

1. Add milk, water, honey, chia seeds, arrowroot, cinnamon, and salt to the crock-pot. Mix well.
2. Lay the slices of apple over this milk mixture.
3. Mix together the ingredients of the topping in a bowl. Sprinkle this mixture over the layer of apples.
4. Set the crock-pot on Low for 4 hours or High for 2 hours.
5. When done, let it stand for a while to set. Sprinkle raisins and walnuts and serve warm or chill and serve cold.

Conclusion

I hope the recipes in this book allowed you to explore the world of slow cooking! Once you know how it works, you could even try to make up and experiment recipes of your own. Slow cooking is easy, relaxing and fun to try out. *And* you get to have time off from the kitchen while the cooker does its job! Leave that soup to simmer while you go work out tomorrow's meeting's agenda or get the kids to finish their homework – that'll definitely take hours!

I hope you found this book informative and instructive!

Part – 2

Introduction

Chicken consumption per capita has been increasing almost every year since the 1960's, or ever since food consumption has been properly monitored. New ingredients may be introduced in the market, fancier restaurants may have popped up at every corner of the street, but humans' cravings for chicken remain the same, if not increased. Chicken can easily be touted as the ultimate favorite when it comes to the preferences of meat lovers. Hence, meal creators too are more focused on making this world favorite all the more delectable, juicier and easier to cook.

People have one common complaint with meals prepared on the slow cooker- all the meals tend to taste the same. It is like saying every pizza tastes the same simply because each one contains dough, cheese and tomato sauce. The fact is, you aren't experimenting enough. This book will definitely bring out the slow cooker meal creator in you.

This book is a collection of recipes that have utilized the convenience and flavor enhancing methodology of the slow cooker to create meals that are small meaty wonders of their own. When paired with the slow cooker, chicken recipes become relentlessly appetizing. So it is just about time you took the slow cooker out of the garage and allowed it to become the star appliance in your kitchen by creating wonders day after day.

Introduction to Slow Cookers

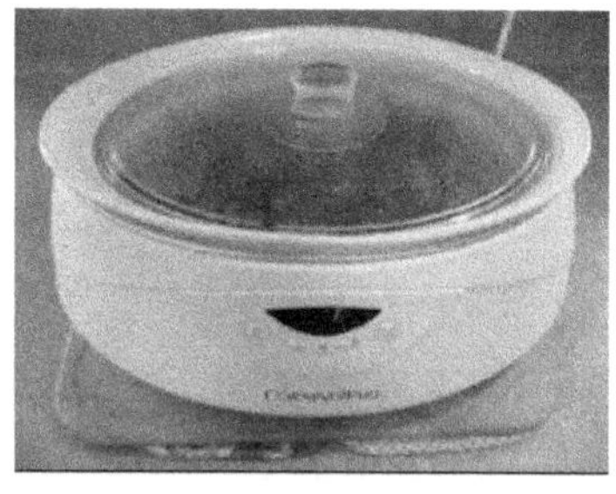

Slow Cooker or Crock-Pot as it is generally known is a lidded oval or round cooking pot which is made from porcelain or glazed ceramic with a metal housing containing the electric heat element. The lid is most commonly glass.

All you need to do is assemble the ingredients in the morning and switch the cooker on. You can easily go about doing your days work, and by the time you are back, your meal would be hot and ready to be devoured. Slow cookers usually come with two or more temperature settings and use very little energy, which means it wouldn't weigh much on your electricity bill or heat up the kitchen the way your oven does, thus limiting any fire hazards.

Slow cookers come in various shapes and sizes ranging from tiny 1-cup slow cookers to larger sizes that can easily cook meals for a family of 4 or even 6. Slow cookers have evolved from simple settings of low and high temperature. Today they come with sophisticated controls that allow you to delay cooking time, keep the food warm once cooked and different programmed settings for cooking specific dishes.

Why Cook in a Slow Cooker?

Slow cooker sales are booming all over. More and more people are opting for these small yet powerful devices to bring convenience and healthy eating back in their life. Nothing is better than coming home to a ready to eat steaming casserole or stew sitting on the kitchen counter.

Meals prepared in the slow cooker are easy on the pocket, easier to cook and the appliance easiest to use. That's a lot of easy in your lifestyle that you can almost get addicted to. But that's not the end. Cooking in the slow cooker has various other benefits also that have been stated below:

1. Tougher cuts of meat become tender more easily in the slow cooker due to condensation. So you can easily purchase cheaper cuts of meat and yet

get full flavor and create tastier meals using less expensive cuts.

2. Vegetables absorb relatively more spices and stocks in the slow cooker, giving them fuller flavors.

3. You can easily adjust the temperature and time on the slow cooker so you don't have to continuously monitor the cooking.

4. Slow cookers are known to prepare meals in 8 to 10 hours, which may be true for some specific meals, but slow cookers today can prepare meals much faster.

5. Slow cooker recipes can be created using limited ingredients thus reduce further cost as well as less preparation time and mess.

6. Don't mistake the multi-cookers for slow cookers, the former have heat elements only at the bottom which can easily burn the dishes.

Slow Cooker Cooking Tips

Following are a list of tried and tested cooking tips to cook the juiciest and most flavorful dishes every time:

1. Fill the slow cooker with about ¾ or preferably ½ of ingredient for best results.
2. Spray the crock with good quality non-stick vegetable spray before you pour in the ingredients. It will prevent the food from sticking to the sides and will make cleaning the equipment very easy.
3. You don't need to add any liquid to the slow cooker. There is no evaporation and so the dishes are cooked with the juices from the ingredients. You might need to add very little liquid in some recipes, in which case it will be mentioned.

4. Every time you take the lid off, the cooking time increases by a good 15 to 20 minutes. So no peeking!

5. You can adjust the seasonings at the end of the cooking. It is quite difficult to assess the flavors and seasoning beforehand. The flavors of herbs become milder during cooking too, so you may need more based on your own liking, so make sure you taste before you serve.

6. Slow cooking takes longer at higher altitudes, so add an extra half an hour of cooking time to each hour of every recipe if you are cooking in higher altitudes.

7. You don't need to add oil to recipes prepared in the slow cooker and you don't need any fat on the meats either. Any fat that's on the meat will not drain away as is the case with normal cooking methods, so make sure you trim most of it away before cooking.

8. The liquid will neither reduce nor thicken as it cooks. If you would like the

broth to be thicker, add a little cornflour at the end (around a teaspoon or two) or roll the meat with seasoned flour before adding it to the slow cooker.

9. Some recipes require browning of some of the ingredients before adding them to the slow cooker. Browning them on the pan will save you a lot of time. However, you can cook them in the slow cooker before adding the rest of the ingredients.

10. Always soak dried beans before cooking. It will reduce the cooking time to 8 hours rather than the standard 18 hours it takes to cook dried beans directly.

11. Slow cooker recipes don't stand well to room temperature, so make sure you refrigerate them immediately once they are cooled off. Don't keep a slow cooker recipe at room temperature for more than two hours.

Standard Cooking Vs. Slow Cooker Cooking

It takes longer for a dish to cook in a slow cooker. But what's the difference like really? Following chart shows the usual time difference.

If A Dish Usually Takes	On High Speed Cook It For	On Low Speed Cook It For
15-30 minutes	1-2 hours	4-6 hours
30 minutes – 1 hour	2-3 hours	5-7 hours
1-2 hours	3-4 hours	6-8 hours
2-4 hours	4-6 hours	8-12 hours

Measurement Guidelines

It is important that you keep the size of the slow cooker in mind when cooking recipes. If you have to buy just one slow cooker then make sure you purchase a larger model, if you are cooking for more than one person. Preferably purchase at least a 6-quarts model. Most recipes suitable for smaller models can easily be made in the larger pot; however, it is not possible the other way round. Following chart shows measurement equivalents to help you properly measure ingredients:

1 tablespoon (tbsp)	3 teaspoons (tsp)
1 tbsp	1/16 cup
2 tbsp	1/8 cup
2 tbsp + 2 tsp	1/6 cup
5 tbsp + 1tsp	1/3 cup
8 tbsp	½ cup
16 tbsp	1 cup
1 quart	4 cups

Now that you have the basics of cooking in a slow cooker covered, it is time to jump right in and get cooking!

Lunch Recipes

1. Creamy Chicken with Biscuits

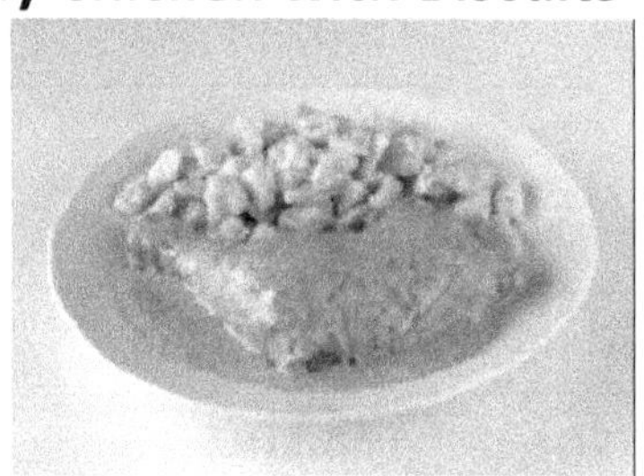

Serves: 6
Slow Cooker Size: 4- to 6- quart
Preparation time: 15 Minutes
Cooking Time: 6 Hours
Ingredients:

- 8 boneless, skinless chicken thighs
- ½ cup chicken broth (preferably low sodium)
- 4 large carrots, cut in 1-inch lengths
- 1 small onion, chopped
- 2 stalks celery, thinly sliced
- ½ tsp poultry seasoning
- ¼ cup all purpose flour
    - 1 cup frozen peas
- ½ cup dry white wine
- ½ cup heavy cream

- Salt and black pepper to taste
- 6 salty biscuits or crackers of your choice

Method:

1. Add flour, carrots, onion to the slow cooker. Place the chicken on top of these ingredients.
2. Season with salt, pepper and poultry seasoning. In the end, add the broth and wine.
3. Cover and cook on high for about 3 hours or on low for about 5 to 6 hours
4. Add the cream, peas and a little more salt if required ten minutes before serving.
5. Serve with biscuits on the bottom and top of the creamy chicken serving.

2. Chicken Tikka Masala

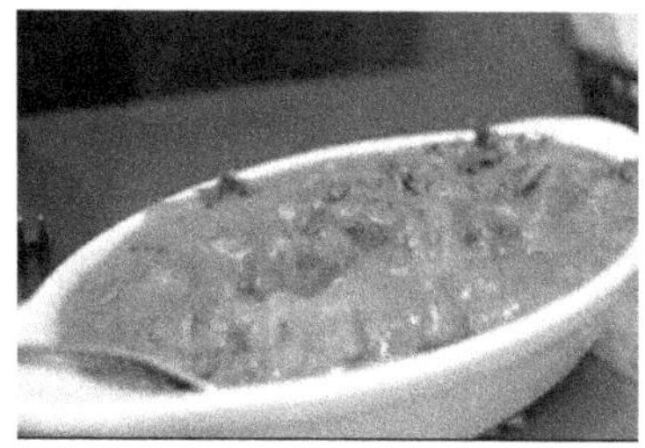

Serves: 4

Slow Cooker Size: 4- to 6- quart

Preparation time: 10 Minutes

Cooking Time: 8 Hours

Ingredient List:

- 8 boneless, skinless chicken thighs
- 1 can of crushed tomatoes, 15 ounce
- 2 cloves of garlic, chopped
- 1 medium sized onion, chopped
- 2 tbsp tomato paste
- Salt and black pepper to taste
- 2 tsp Indian spice blend
    - ½ cup heavy cream
- 1 cup long grain white rice
- 1 tbsp fresh lemon juice
- ¼ cup cilantro leaves, fresh
- ½ cucumber, thinly sliced

1. Add onion, tomatoes, tomato paste, garlic, Indian spice, ¼ tsp pepper, ¾ tsp salt and in the end the chicken to the slow cooker. Cover and cook for 7 to 8 hours on Low or 3 to 4 hours on high speed.
2. Add the cilantro, cucumber, lemon juice and the remaining salt and pepper in a bowl and toss.
3. Cook the rice according to package instructions 20 minutes before the cooking time is up.
4. Once the chicken is cooked, add the cream mix well and serve it with rice and cucumber salad.

3. Chicken and Pasta Soup

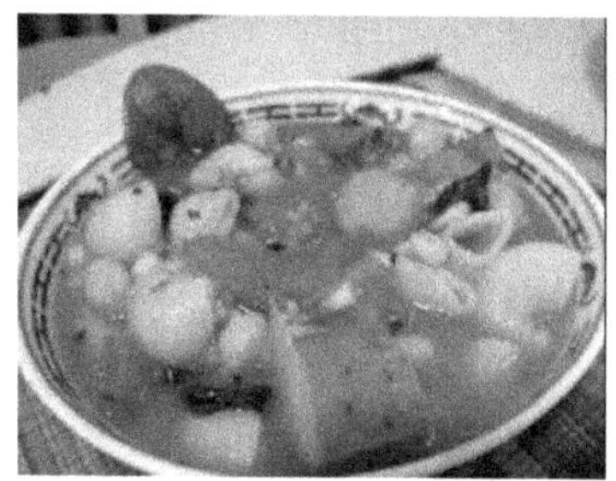

Serves: 6
Slow Cooker Size: 5- to 6- quart
Preparation time: 5 Minutes
Cooking Time: 5 Hours
Ingredients:

- 6 boneless chicken thighs
- ½ cup pasta, opt for alphabet or stellette
- 4 carrots, cut in 1 inch long pieces
- 2 medium potatoes. halved
- 1 medium onion, halved
- 2 bay leaves
- 2 garlic cloves, smashed
    - ¼ cup chopped parsley
- 4 stalks of celery, cut in ½ inch pieces
- Salt and pepper for seasoning

- Crackers for serving (optional)

Method:

1. Add carrots, potato, celery, garlic, onion, 6 cups of water, salt and pepper and chicken to the Crockpot.
2. Cover the pot and cook for 4 to 5 hours on high or 7 to 8 hours on low heat.
3. Transfer the chicken to a bowl 20 minutes before serving and remove the bay leaves and the onion.
4. Shred the chicken.
5. Meanwhile, add the pasta to the slow cooker and cook for about 18 minutes.
6. Once the pasta is ready, add the shredded chicken and parsley in the soup.
7. Serve with crackers (optional).

4. Chicken and Bacon Recipe

Serves: 6
Slow Cooker Size: 4- to 6- quart
Preparation time: 35 Minutes
Cooking Time: 7 Hours

Ingredients:

- 4 pound chicken, cut up
- ½ pound sliced bacon, diced
- ½ pound white mushrooms
- ½ cup dry white wine
- 6 garlic cloves
- 1 cup frozen small white onions (thaw before use)
- 3 sprigs fresh rosemary
    - Salt to taste
- 2 tbsp cornstarch
- ¼ cup water

Method:

1. Cook the bacon on medium-low heat in a large skillet. Transfer the bacon to the slow cooker.

2. Next cook the chicken on the skillet until brown and transfer it to the cooker too.
3. Pour the wine in the skillet to scrape off bacon and chicken bits and then add the contents to the slow cooker.
4. Add onions, mushrooms, rosemary, salt and garlic to the slow cooker and cook for 3 hours on high speed or 6 hours on low speed.
5. Add the sauce from the cooker to the skillet and the rest of the ingredients to a platter. Cook the sauce along with the cornstarch and water until it thickens, or for about 5 minutes.
6. Pour over the bacon and chicken and serve while hot.

5. White Bean and Fennel Recipe

Serves: 6
Slow Cooker Size: 4- to 6- quart
Preparation time: 15 Minutes
Cooking Time: 8 Hours
Ingredients:

- 4 boneless chicken thighs
- 4 carrots
- 8 cups chicken broth (preferably low-sodium)
- 2 stalks celery, chopped
- 1 large onion, chopped
- 1 large fennel bulb, chopped
- 1 cup dried white beans
    - 2 dried bay leaves
- ½ cup small pasta
- Salt and pepper for taste
- Country bread for serving (optional)

Method:

1. Combine carrots, chicken, broth, celery, onion, fennel, beans, salt

and pepper and bay leaves in the slow cooker.

2. Cover and cook for about 4 to 5 hours on high or 7 to 8 hours on low setting.

3. Twenty minutes before serving take out the chicken in a bowl and cook the pasta on high setting.

4. Discard the bay leaves and shred the pasta.

5. Serve the chicken with the pasta soup and bread.

6. Chicken Verde

Serves: 6
Slow Cooker Size: 6- quart
Preparation time: 15 Minutes
Cooking Time: 4 Hours
Ingredients:

- 6 bone-in chicken breast halves, skinned
- 4 jalapeno peppers
- 5 poblano chilies
- 1 large onion, chopped
- 5 garlic cloves, minced
- 5 ½ cups chopped tomatillos
- 1 tbsp sugar
    - 1 can chopped green chilies, drained
- ½ tsp ground cumin
- 1 tbsp canola oil
- Salt and pepper to taste
- 1/3 cup sour cream
- **¼ cup chopped cilantro**

Method:

1. Broil the jalapeno peppers and poblano chilies in the broiler for ten minutes or until charred, turn occasionally. Peel the peppers once cool and cut in half in length. Discard the membrane and seeds. Finely chop the jalapeno peppers and poblano chilies.
2. Add the tomatillos, jalapeno peppers, poblano chilies, onions, sugar, garlic and green chilies in a large bowl.
3. Sprinkle the chicken with pepper and cumin and cook it on medium-high heat in a large skillet until brown on both sides.
4. Add the chicken in the slow cooker along with the tomatillo mixture. Cook on low heat for about 3 and a half hours.
5. Remove the chicken and pour the sauce in a saucepan and bring to a boil. Reduce the heat and cook uncovered until the

liquid is reduced to about 4 cups.

6. Serve the sauce with chicken and garnish with cream and chopped cilantro.

7. Spicy Chicken and Rice

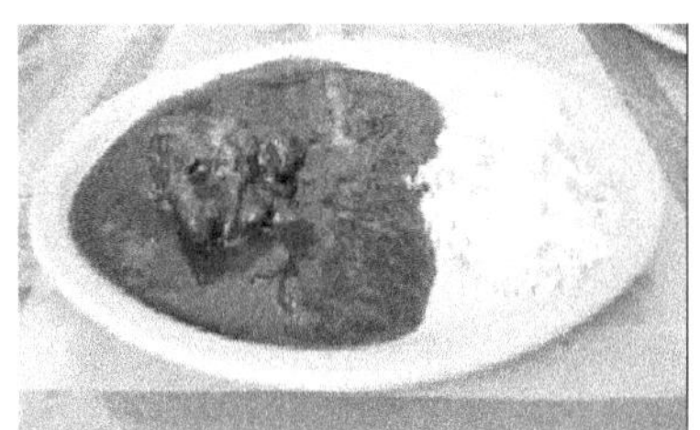

Serves: 6
Slow Cooker Size: 5- quart
Preparation time: 15 Minutes
Cooking Time: 5 Hours
Ingredients:

- 6 skinned chicken thighs
- 1 can stewed tomatoes, chopped
- 6 skinned chicken drumsticks
- 1/3 cup finely chopped onion
- 1 tsp canola oil
- 1/3 cup dry white wine
- ½ tsp salt-free lemon-herb seasoning
    - ¼ tsp salt
- ½ tsp dried Italian seasoning
- 2 garlic cloves, minced
- 3 cups hot cooked rice
- ¼ tsp crushed red pepper

- **¼ tsp dried tarragon**

Method:

1. Trim all the fat from the chicken.
2. Heat a large skillet over medium heat and coat it with the oil.
3. Add chicken to it and cook until browned, turning occasionally, will take around 6 minutes.
4. Add the chicken to the slow cooker.
5. Sautee onion and garlic on the skillet for about two minutes. Add wine and tomatoes next. Remove from heat and add Italian seasoning, lemon-herb seasoning, salt, red pepper and dried tarragon.
6. Add this tomato mixture over the chicken in the slow cooker.
7. Cover and cook for 5 hours on Low setting.
8. Serve with cooked rice.

8. Pulled Chicken Sandwiches

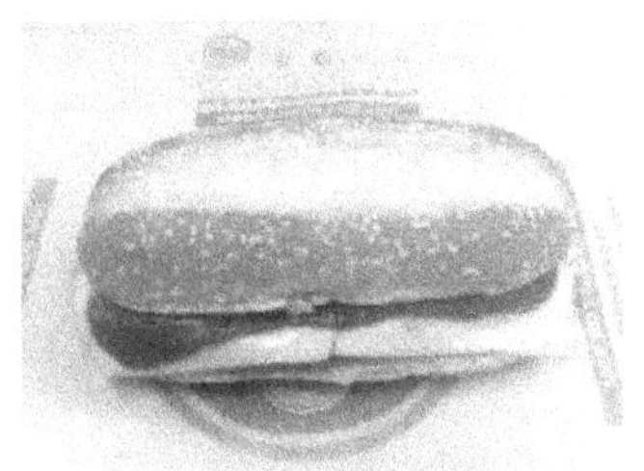

Serves: 8
Slow Cooker Size: 4- quart
Preparation time: 15 Minutes
Cooking Time: 4 Hours
Ingredients:

- 4 skinless, boneless chicken breasts, halved
- 3 cups thinly sliced onion
- 1 cup ketchup
- 1 tsp canola oil
- 2 tbsp cider vinegar
- 1 tbsp Dijon mustard
- 2 tbsp molasses
- ½ tsp garlic powder
- 1 tsp onion powder
- ½ tsp hot sauce

- 1 tsp ground cumin
- 8 whole-wheat burger buns

2 slices of cheese

Method:

1. Add the onions in the slow cooker.
2. Heat a large skillet and add oil to it. Cook the chicken in the skillet until golden brown on both sides, around 6-7 minutes.
3. Add the chicken over the onions in the slow cooker.
4. Add ketchup with the rest of the ingredients (except the buns) and pour over the chicken.
5. Cook on Low setting for 4 hours.
6. Remove the chicken from the cooker when fully cooked and shred it using two forks.
7. Mix the shredded chicken in the sauce.
8. Toast the buns.
9. Add about ¾ cup of chicken mixture to the bottom bun and then cover with the top bun.

Sweet Chicken Thighs

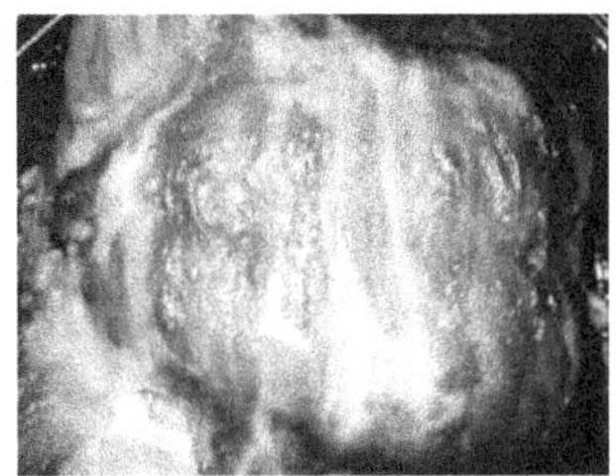

Serves: 6

Slow Cooker Size: 4- quart

Preparation time: 15 Minutes

Cooking Time: 3 Hours

Ingredients:

- 2 pounds skinless, boneless chicken thighs
- Cooking spray
- 1 cup pineapple juice
- Salt and pepper to taste
- 2 tbsp light brown sugar
- 3 tbsp water
- 3 tbsp sliced green onions
- 2 tbsp cornstarch
- 2 tbsp lower-sodium soy sauce
- 1 tbsp olive oil
- 3 cups cooked rice

Method:

1. Sprinkle salt and pepper on the chicken.
2. Heat oil in a large skillet and cook chicken on the skillet for about 3 minutes on each side, or until browned.
3. Transfer the chicken to the slow cooker.
4. Add the pineapple juice to the skillet to scrape off chicken scraping from the pan. Remove the skillet from pan and add soy sauce and brown sugar.
5. Pour this mixture over the chicken and cook for about 2 hours and 45 minutes on Low setting.
6. Transfer only the chicken on to a platter and increase the heat to High on the slow cooker.
7. Mix 3 tbsp of water and cornstarch in a bowl and add this to the sauce in the slow cooker. Mix well and cook for about 2-3 minutes, or until the

sauce thickens. Be sure to constantly stir while the sauce cooks.

8. Serve with a serving of rice topped with the chicken thighs and sauce. Sprinkle with green onions.

Chicken Enchilada

Serves: 8
Slow Cooker Size: 5- quart
Preparation time: 20 Minutes
Cooking Time: 2 Hours
Ingredients:

- 2 cups rotisserie chicken breast
- 1 tsp canola oil
- ½ cup chopped seeded chili
- 1 can no-salt added diced tomatoes
- Cooking spray
- 1 cup frozen baby corn
- 1 cup chopped onion
    - 2 garlic cloves, minced
- 1 ½ tsp chipotle chili powder
- Cilantro sprigs
- 2 cups shredded cheddar cheese
- 5 corn and flour tortillas
    - 1 can tomato sauce with garlic, basil and oregano
- 1 can black beans, rinse and drained

Method:

1. Heat a large skillet over medium heat.
2. Heat oil and add poblano chili, garlic and onion and cook until the vegetables are tender, around 6 minutes.
3. Add tomatoes, tomato sauce and chili powder to the skillet and blend well.
4. Blend the tomato mixture in the blender until almost smooth, blend in two batches to avoid overflow.
5. Coat the slow cooker with cooking spray and add about 3 tbsp of the tomato mixture to it.
6. Combine the rest of the mixture with corn, beans and chicken.
7. Place a tortilla over the sauce in the slow cooker and pour about 1 cup chicken mixture on top. Sprinkle it with 1/3 cup of cheddar cheese and then top it with another tortilla.

8. Repeat with the remaining chicken, cheese and tortillas.
9. Cover and cook on Low for about 2 hours or until the edges are lightly browned.
10. Cut into 8 wedges and garnish with cilantro.

Asian Chicken

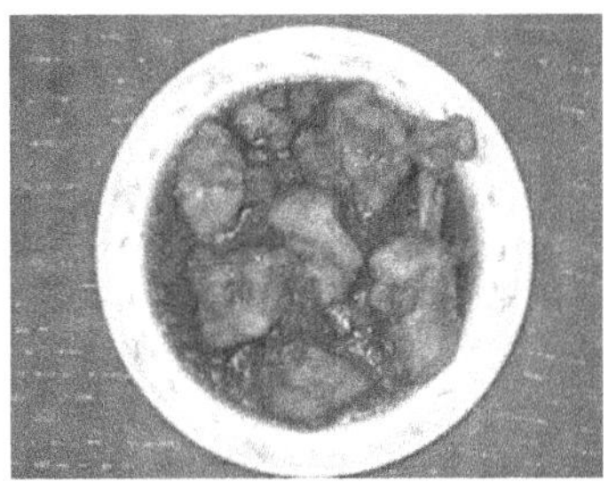

Serves: 8

Slow Cooker Size: 5- quart

Preparation time: 20 Minutes

Cooking Time: 6 Hours

Ingredients:

- 2 pounds boneless chicken thighs, cut into 1 ½ inch cubes
- ½ cup plain yogurt
- 1 can diced tomatoes, drained
- 2 tbsp minced ginger
- 1 onion, coarsely chopped
- 2 tsp curry powder
- 1 large baking potato, peeled and cubed
    - ½ tsp ground cumin
- 1 tsp ground coriander
- ½ tsp crushed red pepper

- 1 tsp salt
- 2 bay leaves
  - 1 cinnamon stick
- 4 cups long-grain brown rice
- ¼ cup fresh cilantro

Method:

1. Sautee the chicken on high heat on a large skillet for about 8 minutes, or until lightly browned.
2. Add the chicken to the slow cooker.
3. Cook the onion in the pan for about 3 minutes. Add ginger, curry powder, cumin, coriander, red pepper and garlic to the onions.
4. Add this mixture over the chicken along with potato, cinnamon stick, tomatoes, bay leaves and salt.
5. Cover and cook on Low setting for 6 hours. Remove the

cinnamon stick and bay leaves once finished.

6. Mix the yogurt in the chicken.

7. Serve the chicken with rice. Sprinkle cilantro for garnish.

12.   Mediterranean Chicken

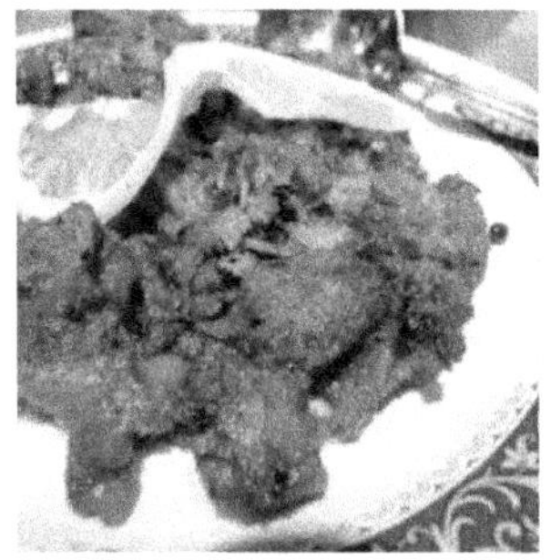

Serves: 6
Slow Cooker Size: 5- quart
Preparation time: 15 Minutes
Cooking Time: 4 Hours
Ingredients:

- 12 bone-in chicken thighs, skinned
- 1 onion, coarsely chopped
- 1 small lemon
- 1 can whole plum tomatoes, coarsely chopped
- 2 tbsp drained capers
- 1 tbsp olive oil
- 12 pitted kalamata olives, halved
- Fresh rosemary and parsley, chopped

Method:

1. Grate, rind and squeeze juice from lemon. Place the rind in a bowl, cover and refrigerate.
2. Add onion, lemon, olives, capers, tomatoes in the slow cooker.
3. Sprinkle pepper on chicken and cook on the skillet until browned from both sides (as prepared in previous recipes). Add the chicken in the slow cooker and cook on Low setting for 4 hours.
4. Place the chicken thighs on a platter.
5. Add the rinds to the sauce and serve over the chicken. Garnish with parsley and rosemary.

Sweet and Sour Chicken

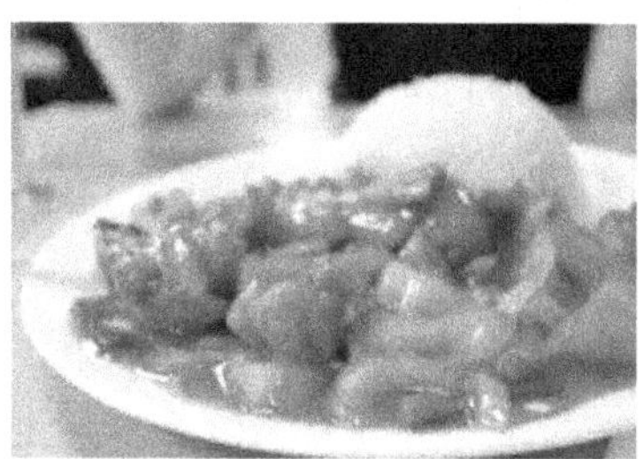

Serves: 6

Slow Cooker Size: 5- 6- quart

Preparation time: 20Minutes

Cooking Time: 6 Hours

Ingredients:

- 4 chicken leg quarters
- 2 tsp ground cumin
- 3 garlic cloves, minced
- 1 can diced tomatoes
- 3 inch fresh ginger, peeled and sliced
- 1 tbsp extra-virgin olive oil
- Salt and pepper to taste
    - ½ tsp ground cinnamon
- 1 medium onion, cut in small wedges
- ½ cup raisins

Method:

1. Combine cinnamon, salt, cumin, pepper in a zip-top bag and mix, then chicken and toss to coat.
2. Heat a large skillet and cook until browned on both sides, around 6 minutes.
3. Place garlic, onion and ginger in the slow cooker. Add the chicken, tomatoes with liquid and raisins.
4. Cover and cook for about 6 hours on Low or 3 ½ hours on high.
5. Serve with rice or bread.

Chicken and Orange

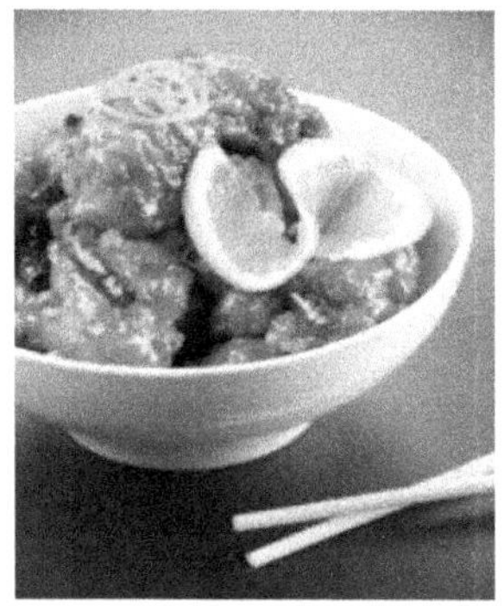

Serves: 4

Slow Cooker Size: 4- to 6- quart

Preparation time: 15 Minutes

Cooking Time:4 Hours

Ingredients:

- 4 skinless chicken thighs
- ½ cup orange marmalade
- ½ cup orange juice
- 1 clove garlic, minced
- ¼ cup soy sauce
- Flour for dredging
- 2 tbsp ketchup
- **2 cups boiled rice**

Method:

1. Remove all visible fat from the chicken.
2. Roll the chicken in flour until fully coated.
3. Add the chicken to the slow cooker.
4. Combine all the remaining ingredients in a bowl and pour over the thighs.
5. Cover and cook for 4 hours on Low setting.
6. Remove the chicken and sauce and serve with boiled rice.

Chicken and Beans

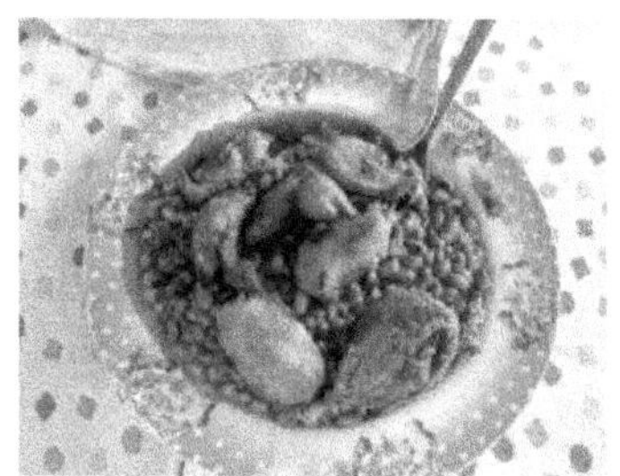

Serves: 4
Slow Cooker Size: 5- to 6- quart
Preparation time: 15 Minutes
Cooking Time: 8 Hours
Ingredients:

- 8 boneless, skinless chicken thighs
- 2 tbsp chopped canned chipotle chilies
- 1 jar mild salsa
- 1 cup dried pinto beans, rinsed
- Salt and pepper to taste
- 2 tbsp all-purpose flour
- 1 medium red onion, chopped
    - ¼ cup sour cream
- ¼ cup chopped fresh cilantro
- 1 red bell pepper, chopped with seeds removed

Method:

1. Add beans, chilies, flour, salsa and 1 cup water in the slow cooker and mix well.
2. Season the chicken with salt and pepper and add that to the salsa mixture.
3. Cover and cook for 8 hours.
4. Remove the chicken and shred in large pieces. Add the chicken pieces to the stew and serve topped with cilantro and sour cream.

Dinner Recipes

Chicken with Potato and Carrots

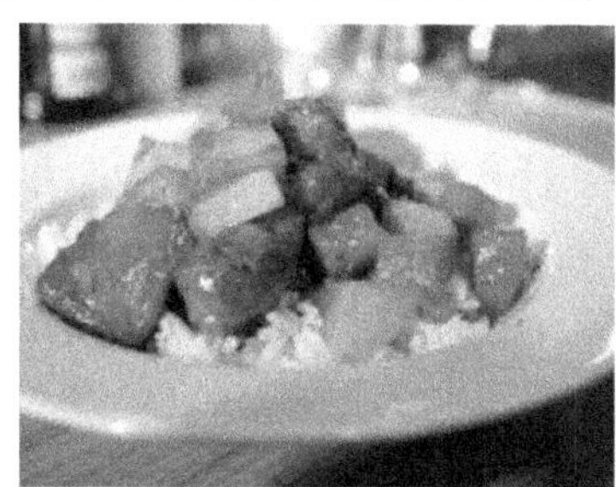

Serves: 6
Slow Cooker Size: 6- quart
Preparation time: 15 Minutes
Cooking Time: 3 ½ Hours
Ingredients:

- 6 chicken thighs, skinned
- 1 onion, vertically sliced
- 2 cups baby carrots
- ½ cup chicken broth
- 6 small red potatoes, cut in thin slices
- 1 tbsp chopped fresh thyme
- 1 tsp paprika

- 1 tsp olive oil
- Salt and pepper to taste
- 1 tsp minced garlic
- ½ cup dry white wine

Method:

1. Add the potatoes, carrots and onions in the slow cooker.
2. In a large bowl combine the chicken broth, salt and pepper, wine, thyme and garlic and mix well. Pour this mixture over the vegetables in the slow cooker.
3. Combine paprika with a little salt and pepper and rub over the chicken. Cook the chicken on a large skillet until browned on both sides, about 6 minutes.
4. Place the chicken on top of the vegetables. Cover and cook on Low setting for about 3 ½ hours or until chicken is fully cooked.
5. Serve over a bed of rice.

Curried Chicken

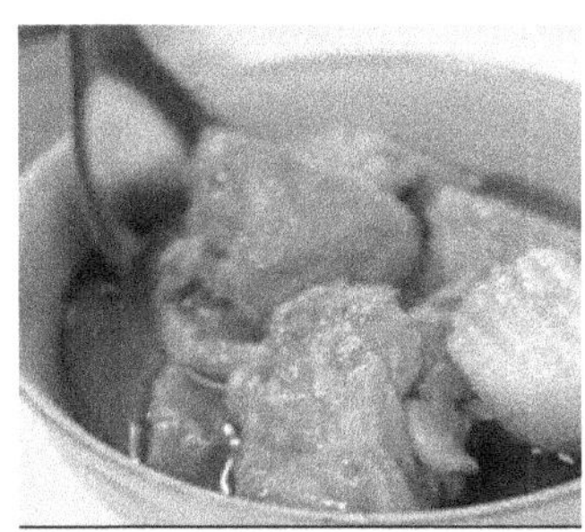

Serves: 6
Slow Cooker Size: 4- to 6- quart
Preparation time: 15 Minutes
Cooking Time: 8 Hours
Ingredients:

- 10 boneless, skinless chicken thighs
- 1/3 cup tomato paste
- 1 tbsp grated fresh ginger
- 1 ½ cup white rice, cooked
- 2 scallions thinly sliced
- 1 tsp ground cumin
- 4 cloves garlic, chopped
    - 1 tbsp fresh ginger
- 2 tbsp curry powder

- 1 onion, chopped
- Salt and pepper to taste
- ½ cup Greek yogurt

Method:

1. Whisk ginger, ¾ cup water, tomato paste, garlic, cumin and curry powder together. Add onion and blend well. Add this paste to the slow cooker.
2. Season the chicken with salt and pepper and place on the paste in the slow cooker.
3. Cover and cook on Low setting for 8 hours.
4. Add yogurt and a little more salt, if desired right before serving.
5. Serve with rice and top with sliced scallions.

Soy Braised Chicken

Serves: 4
Slow Cooker Size: 5- to 6- quart
Preparation time: 10 Minutes
Cooking Time: 8 Hours
Ingredients:

- 8 skinless chicken thighs
- 2 medium sized onions, sliced
- 1/3 cup apple cider vinegar
- 1 tbsp brown sugar
- Salt and pepper to taste
- 1 tsp paprika
- 1 cup white rice, cooked
    - 4 garlic cloves, smashed
- 1/3 cup soy sauce
- 1 large head bok choy (Chinese cabbage), cut in small strips
- 2 scallions, thinly sliced
- 1 tbsp brown sugar

Method:

1. Combine vinegar, soy sauce, garlic, onions, brown sugar,

pepper and bay leaf in the slow cooker. Add the chicken on top and sprinkle paprika.

2. Cover and cook for 8 hours on Low setting, or for 4 hours on High if preparing for lunch.
3. Turn the heat on High, if cooking on slow, in the last ten minutes.
4. Fold the bok choy in the chicken gently and cook for another 5 minutes.
5. Serve with rice and garnish with scallions.

Surf and Turf with Shrimp and Chicken

Serves: 8
Slow Cooker Size: 6- quart
Preparation time: 15 Minutes
Cooking Time: 5 Hours
Ingredients:

- 4 skinless, boneless chicken thighs cut in small pieces
- 4 skinless, boneless chicken breasts, cut in small pieces
- 2 cups chopped onion
- 1 cup chopped celery
- 1 cup chopped green pepper
- 2 garlic cloves, minced
- ½ tsp dried thyme
    - 4 ounces turkey kielbasa (sausage), cut in thin slices
- 2 tsp Cajun seasoning
- ¼ tsp Spanish smoked paprika
- 1 can fat-free chicken broth
- 1 pound medium shrimp, peeled and deveined
    - 1 tbsp hot sauce
- 2 tbsp chopped parsley
- 2 ½ cups long-grain rice, cooked
- 2 cans diced tomatoes with green peppers and onions, undrained

Method:

1. Heat a large skillet on high heat and cook the chicken on both sides until lightly browned, around 4 minutes. Add the chicken to the slow cooker
2. Add celery, bell pepper, onion and garlic in the skillet and cook until tender, around 4 minutes.
3. Add the turkey kielbasa, onion mixture, Cajun seasoning, dried thyme, tomatoes, paprika and chicken broth in the slow cooker.
4. Cover and cook on Low setting for 5 hours.
5. Add the cooked rice and the remaining ingredients in the slow cooker and cook on High setting for about 15 minutes, or until the shrimps are cooked.

Spicy Chicken Stew

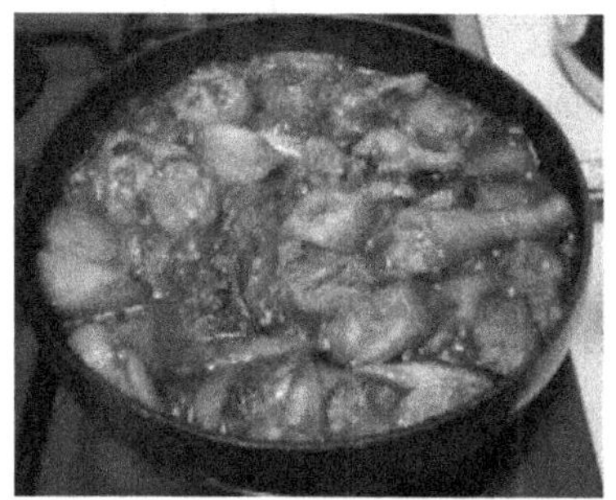

Serves: 6
Slow Cooker Size: 5- quart
Preparation time: 10 Minutes
Cooking Time: 4 Hours
Ingredients:

- 4 skinless, boneless chicken thighs
- 1 pound skinless, boneless chicken breast
- 2 baking potatoes, peeled and cut in cubes
- 2 celery stalks, chopped
- 1 onion, roughly chopped
- 1 package frozen whole-kernel corn
- 2 carrots, peeled and cubed

- 2 ½ cups low-sodium chicken broth
- 2 garlic gloves, minced
- 1 ½ tsp ground cumin
- 1 cup bottled salsa
- 1 tsp chili powder
- Salt and pepper to taste
- 4 corn tortillas, cut in strips

Method:

1. Add potatoes, corn, celery, carrots, onion and garlic in the slow cooker. Add salsa on top along with pepper, cumin and chili powder. Add the chicken on top of the vegetables. Pour the broth on top.
2. Cover and cook on High setting for 4 hours.
3. Remove the chicken and shred it using forks.
4. Place the rest of the vegetables and broth in a serving dish. Add shredded chicken and the tortilla strips in the stew.

21.   *Chicken Mole*

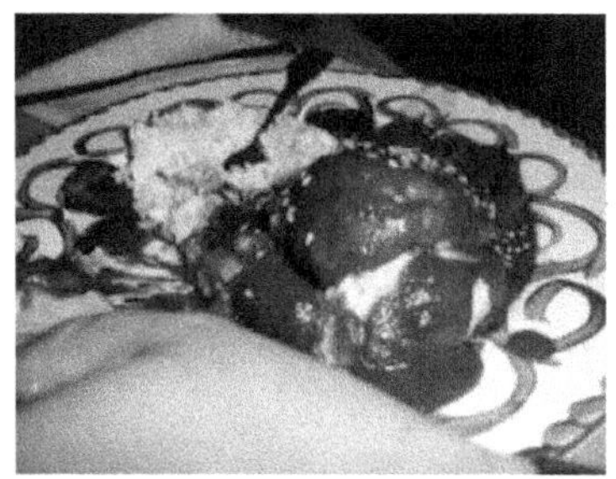

Serves: 6
Slow Cooker Size: 5- 6- quart
Preparation time: 15 Minutes
Cooking Time: 4 Hours 15 Minutes
Ingredients:

- 12 boneless, skinless chicken thighs
- 1 can whole tomatoes
- 2 dried ancho chiles, stemmed
- 1 medium onion, roughly chopped
- 1 large chipotle chile in adobo sauce
- Salt to taste
- ¼ cup raisins
    - ½ cup sliced almonds, toasted
- 3 garlic cloves, peeled and smashed
- ¾ tsp ground cumin

- ½ cup bittersweet chocolate, finely chopped
- 3 tbsp extra-virgin olive oil
  - ½ tsp ground cinnamon
- 2 cups boiled white rice

Method:

1. Season the chicken thighs with salt and place them in the slow cooker.
2. Puree the rest of the ingredients (except rice) in the blender. Add this mixture to the blender.
3. Cover and cook on Low setting for 8 hours or 4 hours on High if preparing for lunch.
4. Serve on top of a bed of rice.

Chicken with Garlic and Couscous

Serves: 4

Slow Cooker Size: 5- 6- quart

Preparation time: 25 Minutes

Cooking Time: 4 Hours

Ingredients:

- 1 whole chicken, cut in 8 pieces
- 1 medium onion, thinly sliced
- Salt and pepper to taste
- 1 tbsp extra-virgin olive oil
- 1 cup dry white wine
- 6 garlic cloves, halved
- 1 cup couscous, cooked according to package instructions
  - 1/3 cup all-purpose flour
- 2 tsp dried thyme

Method:

1. Season the chicken with salt and pepper and cook it on a large skillet until golden brown on all sides. Preferably cook in batches to ensure it is properly browned,

should take about 4 minutes for each batch.

2. Add thyme, garlic and onion in the slow cooker. Add salt and pepper for seasoning. Layer the chicken on top of the onions in the slow cooker with skin side up. Be sure to make a tight layer.

3. Add wine and flour in a small bowl and whisk until blended. Add this to the slow cooker too.

4. Cover and cook on Low for 7 hours or for 3 ½ hours on High setting.

5. Serve the chicken over couscous.

Mexican Stew

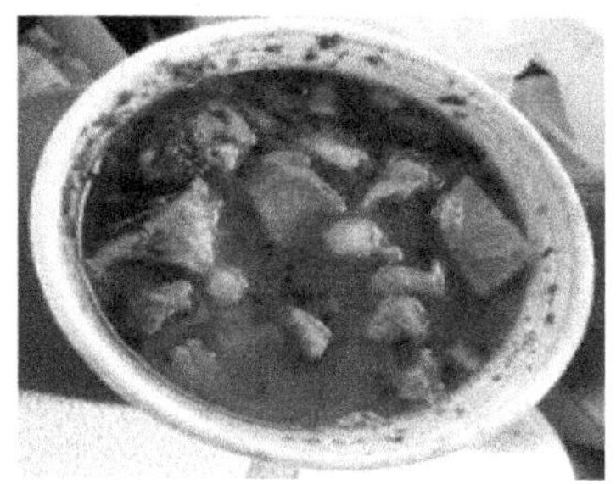

Serves: 4
Slow Cooker Size: 5- quart
Preparation time: 20 Minutes
Cooking Time: 7 Hours
Ingredients:

- 4 skinless, boneless chicken breasts
- 1 tbsp extra virgin olive oil
- 1 medium onion, finely chopped
- ½ tsp dark brown sugar
- 1 (400g) can chopped tomatoes
- 1 small red onion, sliced into rings
- 1 tsp chipotle paste
- **4 corn tortillas**

Method:

1. Heat oil in a small skillet and sauté the onions. Add the onions along with the rest of the ingredients to the slow cooker.
2. Cover and cook on Low setting for 7 hours.
3. Remove the chicken and shred using two forks. Put the chicken back in the sauce. Serve with tortillas.

Chicken Stew with White Wine

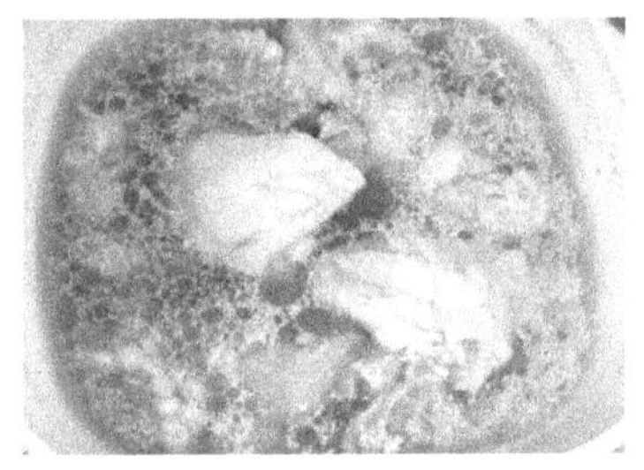

Serves: 4
Slow Cooker Size: 6- quart
Preparation time: 15 Minutes
Cooking Time: 4 Hours
Ingredients:

- 1 pound skinless, boneless chicken breasts, cubed
- 1 cup chicken broth
- 3 tbsp olive oil

- 1 pound cremini mushrooms, quartered
- 2 onions, sliced
- 2 Portobello mushrooms, sliced
- 1 cup dry white wine
- Salt and pepper to taste

Method:

1. Heat oil in a large skillet and cook the chicken until browned on both sides, around 5 minutes.
2. Add onions and mushroom in a saucepan and sate until both release their juices and turn golden brown. Be sure to continuously stir.
3. Add the onions and mushrooms to the slow cooker. Place chicken on top and season with salt and pepper.
4. Cover and cook on Low setting for 4 hours, or until the chicken is tender.

25.   Chicken Stroganoff

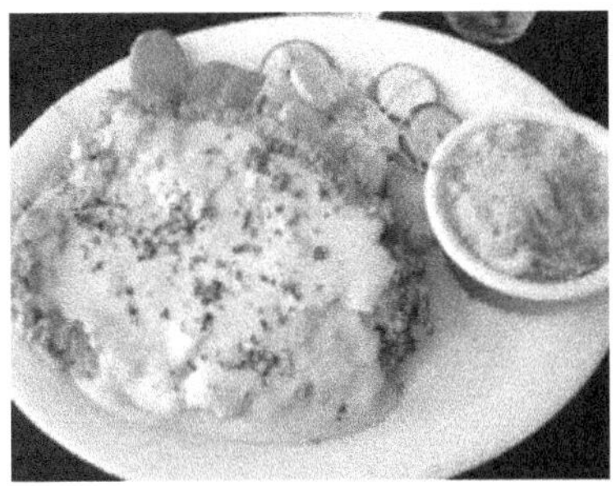

Serves: 4
Slow Cooker Size: 5- quart
Preparation time: 15 Minutes
Cooking Time: 5 Hours 30 Minutes
Ingredients:

- 4 skinless, boneless chicken breast halves, cubed
- 1 package cream cheese, 8 ounce
- 1 can condensed cream of chicken soup
- 1/8 cup margarine
- 1 package dry Italian-style salad dressing mix

Method:

1. Add dressing mix, margarine and chicken in the slow cooker.

2. Cover and cook for 5 hours on Low setting.

3. Add the rest of the ingredients to the chicken and cook for another half hour on High setting.

26.   *BBQ Chicken*

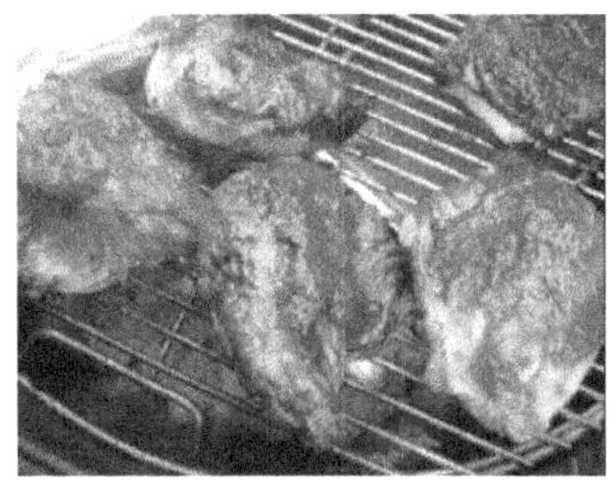

Serves: 4
Slow Cooker Size: 6- quart
Preparation time: 5 Minutes
Cooking Time: 4 Hours
Ingredients:

- 3 large skinless chicken breasts, and bone-in
- 3 tbsp brown sugar
- 2 tbsp all purpose steak seasoning
- 1 cup BBQ sauce

Method:

1. Make 4 large balls from foil and fit them to the bottom of your slow cooker.

2. Season the chicken with brown sugar and steak seasoning
3. Place the chicken breasts on the foil balls in the slow cooker and pour the BBQ sauce over them.
4. Cover and cook on High setting for 4 hours or until the chicken is cooked.
5. Serve the chicken on a platter with remaining juices from the slow cooker poured over it.
6. You can also shred the chicken, mix it with the juices and serve with rice.

Lemon Chicken

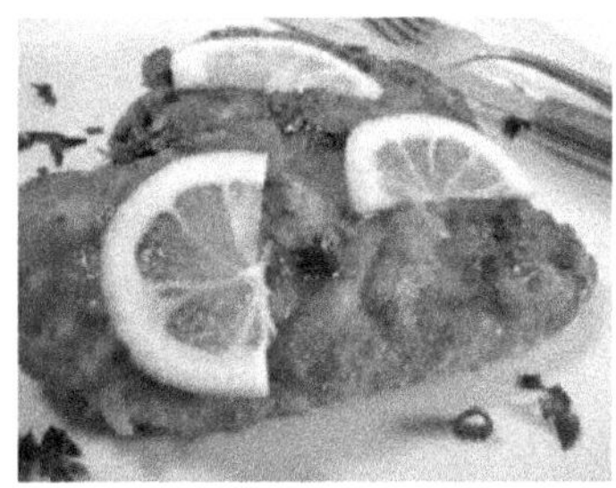

Serves: 8
Slow Cooker Size: 5- 6- quart
Preparation time: 15 Minutes
Cooking Time: 6 Hours

Ingredients:

- 12 boneless, skinless chicken thighs
- 1 cup low sodium chicken broth
- Salt and pepper to taste
- 1 lemon sliced,
- 2 tbsp olive oil, divided
- ¾ cup pitted green olives
- ¼ cup flour or cornstarch
- 2 tbsp lemon juice, freshly squeezed

Method:

1. Heat oil in a large skillet over medium heat and cook the chicken until browned on both sides, around six minutes. Preferably do it in batches.
2. Add the chicken to the slow cooker and cover with lemon slices.
3. Combine flour, cumin and juice and whisk until combined. Pour the broth over the chicken and top with olives and black pepper for seasoning.
4. Cover and cook for 6 hours on Low setting, or until well cooked.

Jamaican Chicken

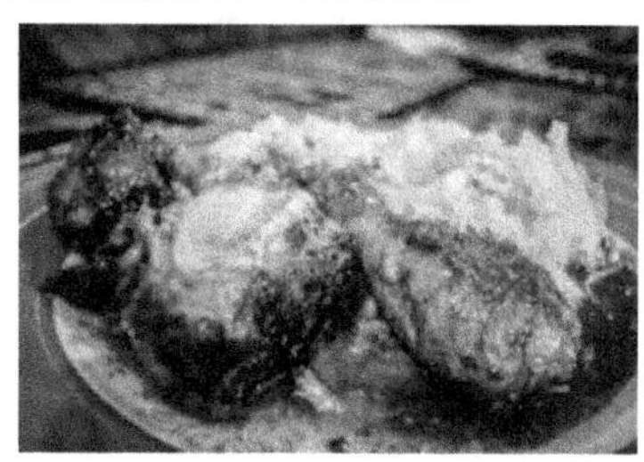

Serves: 8

Slow Cooker Size: 6- quart

Preparation time: 15 Minutes

Cooking Time: 3 Hours

Ingredients:

- 8 boneless skinless chicken breast halves
- 2 tbsp rice vinegar
- 2 tsp jerk seasoning
- ½ cup light brown sugar
- 1 ½ cups mango nectar
- 2 tbsp dark corn syrup

Method:

1. Add nectar, corn syrup, sugar, jerk seasoning and rice vinegar in the

slow cooker and mix well. Add the chicken and coat it in the sauce.

2. Cover and cook on High setting for 3 hours.

Tea Smoked Chicken Legs

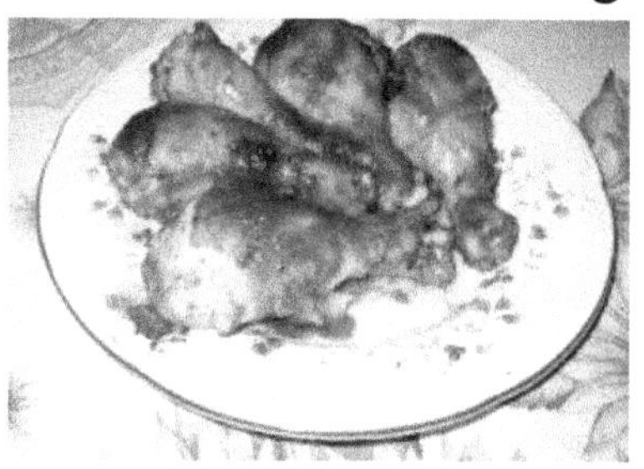

Serves: 6
Slow Cooker Size: 5- to 7- quart
Preparation time: 5 Minutes
Cooking Time: 5 Hours
Ingredients:

- 6 skinless chicken legs
- 2 cups chicken broth
- 8 bags black tea
- 1 cinnamon stick
- 4 slices ginger
- ¼ cup hoisin sauce
- ½ cup soy sauce

Method:

1. Boil the chicken broth in a saucepan and add the tea bags, cinnamon and

ginger. Remove from heat and allow the broth to cool. Strain and mix hoisin and soy sauce.

2. Brush a little sauce on the legs. Pour the rest in the slow cooker. Add the chicken legs.

3. Cover and cook for 5 hours, basting the chicken 3 or 4 times during cooking.

30.Chicken Corn Soup

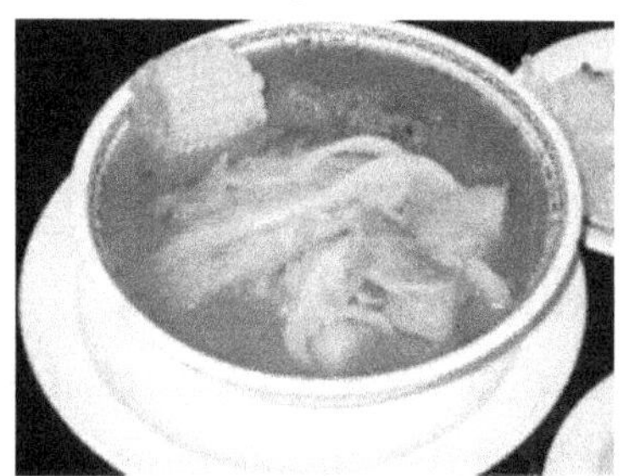

Serves: 6

Slow Cooker Size: 4- to 6- quart

Preparation time: 15 Minutes

Cooking Time: 8-9 Hours

Ingredients:

- 1 pound boneless skinless chicken breast, cubed
- ½ tsp minced garlic
- 12 ounce cream style corn
- ½ cup chopped celery
- ¾ cup sliced carrots
- 1 cup chopped onion
- Salt and pepper to taste
    - 2 medium potatoes, cubed
- 12 ounces frozen corn
- 2 cups low sodium chicken broth

Method:

1. Combine all the ingredients in the slow cooker.
2. Cover and cook for 8 hours.

Quick Slow Cooker Recipes

Chicken with Figs
Serves: 6
Slow Cooker Size: 5- 7- quart
Preparation time: 15 Minutes
Cooking Time: 2 Hours
Ingredients:

- 6 boneless skinless chicken breast halves
- 2 tbsp vegetable oil
- Salt and freshly ground black pepper to taste
- ½ cup balsamic biegar
- ½ cup low-sodium chicken broth
- ½ cup Ruby Port
- 1 6 dried figs
- 1 tsp dried thyme

Method:

1. Season the chicken with salt and pepper and cook it on a large skillet until both sides are golden brown, around 6 minutes.
2. Transfer the chicken to a slow cooker.
3. Scrape up the browns from the skillet using port and vinegar and pour it over the chicken.
4. Add the remaining ingredients.
5. Cover and cook on High setting for 2 hours.

Crockpot Pesto Chicken Thighs

Serves: 8
Slow Cooker Size: 6- quart
Preparation time: 15 Minutes
Cooking Time: 3 Hours
Ingredients:

- 8 boneless chicken thighs
- 1 package seasoning mix
- ½ cup chicken broth
- 6 ounce jar of pesto

Method:

1. Place chicken thighs, ranch dressing, pesto and chicken broth in the slow cooker.
2. Cover and cook for two and a half hours on High setting, or until the chicken is cooked.

Sesame and Honey Wings

Serves: 4
Slow Cooker Size: 4- quart
Preparation time: 15 Minutes
Cooking Time: 2 Hours
Ingredients:

- 1 1/2 pounds chicken wings
- 1/8 cup oil
- Salt and pepper to taste
- 1 cup honey
- ½ cup soy sauce
- ¼ cup catsup
- 1 clove garlic, minced
- Sesame seeds for garnish

Method:

1. Place the wings in broiler pan and sprinkle salt and pepper on top. Place the pan about 5 inches under broiler and broil for 7 minutes on each side or until the chicken is golden.

2. Move the wings to the slow cooker
   and add the remaining ingredients,
   except the sesame seeds.
3. Cover and cook for 2 hours on High
   setting.

Tuscan Soup

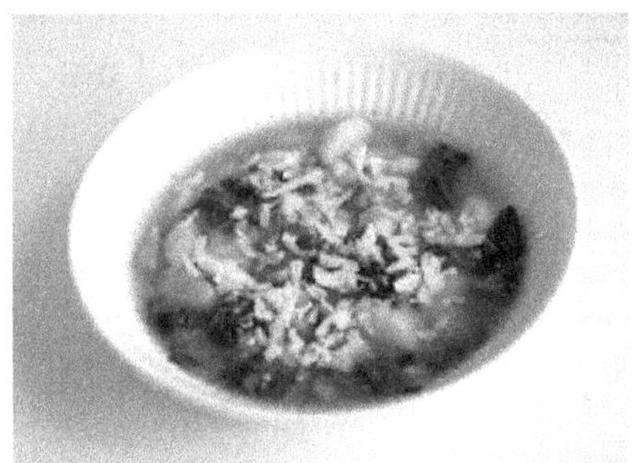

Serves: 4

Slow Cooker Size: 5- quart

Preparation time: 15 Minutes

Cooking Time: 3 Hours

Ingredients:

- 1 pound boneless, skinless chicken thighs, cut in small pieces
- 1 cup chopped onion
- Salt and freshly ground black pepper to taste
- 1 can low sodium chicken broth
- 1 can cannellini beans, rinsed and drained
- 3 garlic cloves, minced

- 8 tbsp grated Parmesan cheese
- 1 package fresh baby spinach
- ½ tsp chopped rosemary
- 1 bottle roasted red bell peppers, drained and cut in small pieces
- 2 tbsp tomato paste

Method:

1. Add onions, tomato, beans, broth, bell peppers, salt and pepper, chicken and garlic in the slow cooker.
2. Cover and cook on High setting for an hour. Reduce the heat and then cook for another 2 hours, or until the chicken is fully cooked.
3. Add rosemary and spinach and cook for another 10 minutes on Low.
4. Serve the soup in bowls topped with cheese.

Chicken Cacciatore

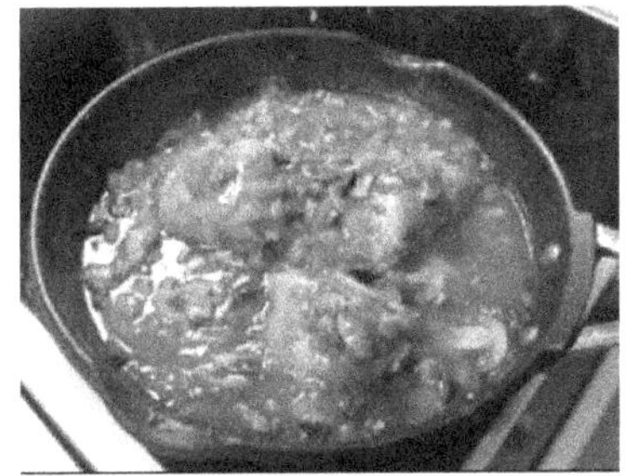

Serves: 8

Slow Cooker Size: 5- quart

Preparation time: 15 Minutes

Cooking Time: 3 Hours

Ingredients:

- 8 bone-in, skinned chicken drumsticks
- 8 bone-in, skinned chicken thighs
- Salt and black pepper to taste
- 2 tbsp minced garlic
- 1 tbsp olive oil
- 1 package mushrooms, quartered
- 1 large onion, sliced
    - 1 red bell pepper, sliced
- 1 green bell pepper, sliced
- 1/3 cup all purpose flour

- 2 tbsp chopped fresh thyme
- 2 tbsp chopped fresh oregano
  - ½ cup red wine
- 1 can whole plum tomatoes, chopped

Method:

1. Season the chicken with salt and pepper and cook on a skillet until lightly browned on both sides, around 6 minutes.
2. Add the chicken to the slow cooker and top it with the mushrooms.
3. Add bell peppers, garlic and onion to a pan and season with salt. Cook the vegetables for 5 minutes on medium heat. Add wine to the vegetables and cook for another minute, scraping the brown bits off. Add oregano, tomatoes, flour and thyme.
4. Add this tomato mixture to the chicken in the slow cooker.
5. Cover and cook for 3 hours on High setting.

6. Preferably serve with fettuccine.

Chicken Ginger and Sesame Lunch Special

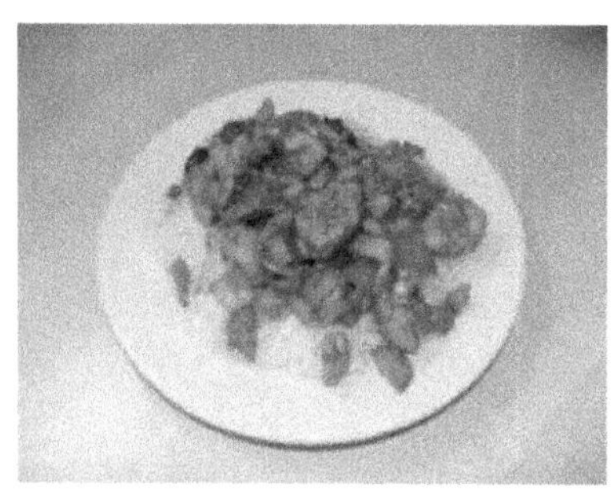

Serves: 4
Slow Cooker Size: 4- quart
Preparation time: 15 Minutes
Cooking Time: 2 ½ Hours
Ingredients:

- 8 bone-in chicken thighs, skinned
- ¼ cup soy sauce
- 5 tsp hoisin sauce
- 1 tbsp sesame oil
- 2 tbsp light brown sugar
- 1 tbsp cornstarch
- 2 tbsp fresh orange juice
    - 2 tsp sesame seeds, toasted

- 1 tbsp cold water
- 2 tbsp sliced green onions
- 1 tbsp minced ginger
- 1 tsp minced garlic

Method:

1. Cook the chicken in batches in a large skillet until golden brown, ideally 5 minutes.
2. Transfer chicken to the slow cooker.
3. Add soy sauce, garlic, brown sugar, hoisin sauce, ginger and orange juice in a medium sized bowl and pour over the chicken.
4. Cover and cook on Low setting for 2 ½ hours or until the chicken is tender. Transfer chicken to the serving platter.
5. Sieve the sauce in the slow cooker and bring it to a boil in over medium heat. Discard the solids. S
6. Combine cornstarch and cold water and pour it in the sauce to make it thick. Cook for another minute and pour the sauce over the chicken.

7. Sprinkle green onions and sesame seed
    on top.

Spinach Stuffed Chicken Breasts

Serves: 6
Slow Cooker Size: 6- 7- quart
Preparation time: 15 Minutes
Cooking Time: 3 Hours
Ingredients:

- 6 boneless skinless breast halves
- 2 tbsp olive oil
- Salt and pepper to taste
- One packet of frozen chopped spinach, defrosted and squeezed dry
- 1 ½ cups chicken broth
- ¼ tsp freshly grated nutmet
- ¼ cup finely chopped shallot
    - ½ cup dry white wine
- 1 cup heavy cream
- ¼ cup finely chopped chives
- One package Boursin cheese, 2-ounce

Method:

1. Place the chicken in plastic wraps and pound until the chicken gets a

uniform thickness. Season it with salt and pepper.

2. Sauté the shallots in oil in a medium sized skillet, for about 2 minutes. Add spinach and cook until wilted. Season with salt, pepper and nutmeg and stir well. Once cool at Boursin cheese.

3. Spread the shallot stuffing on the chicken breasts. Roll up the chicken breasts and tuck sides to enclose the filling.

4. Now lay these seam side down in the slow cooker and pour the wine on top. Use skewers if the rolls aren't properly secured.

5. Cover and cook on high setting for 2 ½ hours.

6. Carefully remove the chicken and cover with foil. Pour the sauce in a saucepan and bring to a boil. Cook for another five minutes or until the sauce is reduced to half. Bring the heat to low and add the cream. Remove from heat and stir in chives.

7. Cu each chicken breast into 4 pieces
    crosswise.

8. Serve the chicken with the sauce.

Chicken and Red Wine Casserole

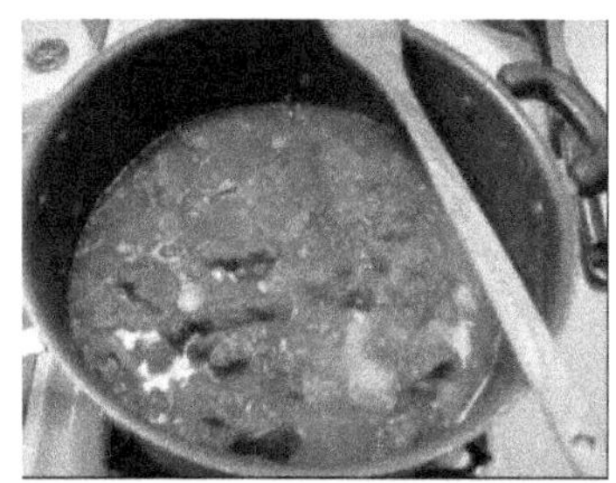

Serves: 6
Slow Cooker Size: 4- quart
Preparation time: 15 Minutes
Cooking Time: 8 Hours
Ingredients:

- 6 bone-in chicken breasts
- 3 tbsp olive oil
- 3 tbsp plain flour
- 3 onions, cut in wedges
- 3 garlic cloves
- 200g smoked bacon lardons
- 300g flat mushrooms, sliced

- 2 tbsp redcurrant sauce
- 1 cup red wine
- 3 strips of orange zest
- 1 cup low-sodium chicken stock
- 2 bay leaves

Method:

1. Season the chicken with salt and pepper and cook on medium heat in a large skillet until lightly browned on both sides, around five minutes.
2. Add the onions and lardons and cook for another 6 minutes. Sprinkle the plain flour and add garlic and cook for another minute. Be sure to keep on stirring to avoid sticking.
3. Add the chicken and bacon along with the remaining ingredients in the slow cooker and cook on Low heat for 8 hours.

Orange Cranberry Chicken

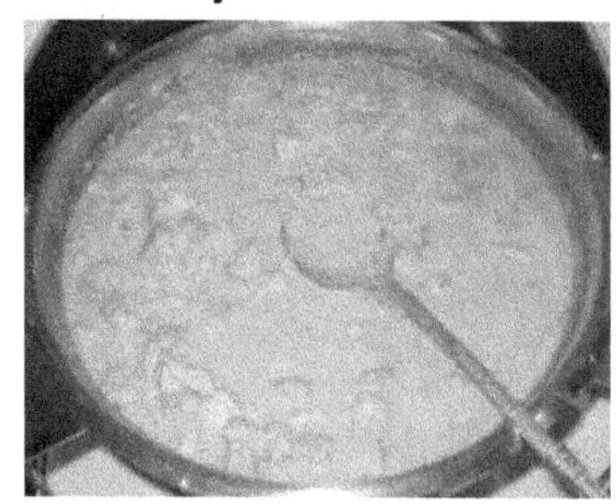

Serves: 6
Slow Cooker Size: 5- quart
Preparation time: 15 Minutes
Cooking Time: 6 Hours
Ingredients:

- 6 skinless, boneless chicken breast halves, cut in small pieces
- 1 cup low-sodium chicken broth
- 1 tbsp margarine
- ¼ cup brown sugar
- 1 tsp chopped ginger
- 1/3 cup reduced-sugar orange marmalade
- 1 tbsp rice vinegar
    - ½ tsp ground cinnamon

- ½ cup dried cranberries

Method:

1. Add all the ingredients, except chicken, in the slow cooker and blend well.
2. Place the chicken on the top, cover and cook on Low setting for 6 hours.
3. Serve with the sauce, preferably with brown rice.

Chicken Pesto Potato

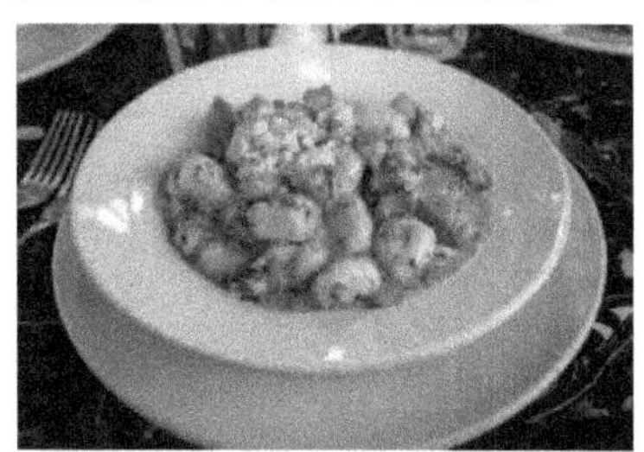

Serves: 4

Slow Cooker Size: 5- quart

Preparation time: 15 Minutes

Cooking Time: 6 Hours

Ingredients:

- 4 skinless, boneless chicken breasts
- 4 tbsp prepared pesto
- 1 ½ tsp olive oil
- 1 tsp lemon pepper seasoning
- ½ cup low-sodium chicken broth
- 4 cups potato pieces, partially cooked in the microwave
- ½ cup chopped red bell pepper

Method:

1. Heat a large nonstick pan and cook the chicken breasts with olive oil until lightly browned on both sides, around 6 minutes.
2. Add the potato pieces to the slow cooker and pour the chicken broth on top.
3. Spread pesto evenly over the top and sprinkle with red pepper. Gently toss the mixture and place the chicken on top.
4. Cover and cook for about 6 hours on Low setting.

Chicken Vegetable Soup with Noodles

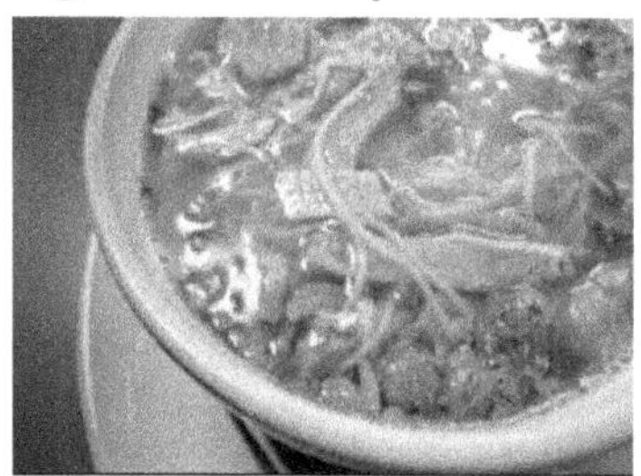

Serves: 6

Slow Cooker Size: 4- to 6- quart

Preparation time: 15 Minutes

Cooking Time: 7 Hours

Ingredients:

- 3 pound chicken
- 2 cups sliced carrots
- 2 cups chopped onion
- 1 cup uncooked egg noodles
- 2 cups celery
- Salt and pepper to taste
- ½ tsp basil
    - 10 ounces frozen peas
- 2 tbsp parsley
- 2 cups water
- ¼ tsp thyme

1. Add all the ingredients in the slow cooker except noodles, place chicken on top of the rest of the ingredients.
2. Cover and cook for 6 hours on Low setting.
3. Add the noodles, cover and cook on High setting for another hour.

42.   Peanut Butter Wings

Serves: 8
Slow Cooker Size: 6- quart
Preparation time: 20 Minutes
Cooking Time: 3-4 Hours
Ingredients:

- 3 pounds chicken wings
- Salt and pepper to taste
- ¼ cup olive oil
- 1 tsp paprika
- ½ cup chicken broth
- 2 tbsp soy sauce
- ¼ tsp hot sauce
    - 2 tsp grated ginger
- ¼ cup brown sugar
- 1 cup smooth peanut butter
- 1 can coconut milk, 14-ounce
- ½ cup roasted peanuts, finely chopped

Method:

1. Put the wings, olive oil, paprika, pepper and salt in a large bowl and mix well until the wings are well

coated. Arrange the wings on a baking sheet and broil in a preheated broiler for about 5 minutes on each side, or until crispy brown.

2. Combine all the remaining ingredients, except peanuts, in a saucepan over medium heat and cook for 2 minutes. Pour the sauce over the wings.

3. Transfer the sauce and the wings in the slow cooker.

4. Cover and cook for 3 hours.

5. Serve with a garnish of peanuts.

Slow Cooker Recipes For Kids

Chili Chicken Tacos

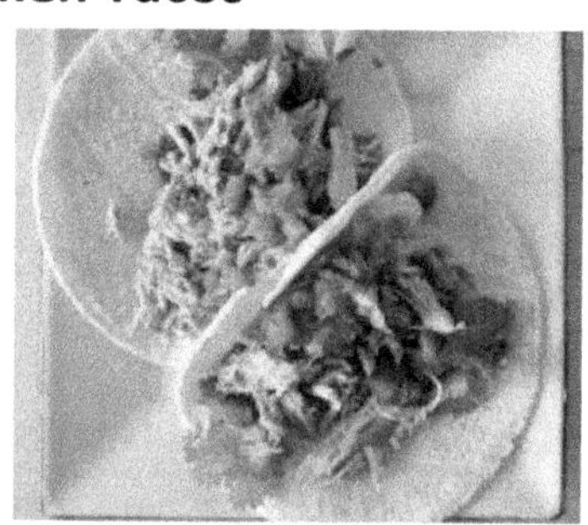

Serves: 4
Slow Cooker Size: 4- quart
Preparation time: 15 Minutes
Cooking Time: 4 Hours
Ingredients:

- 6 boneless, skinless chicken thighs
- ½ cup prepared tomato salsa
- 4 garlic cloves
- 1 tbsp chili powder
- 2 tbsp chopped canned chipotle chiles in adobo

- Salt and pepper to taste
- 8 hard corn taco shells
- **1 tbsp chili powder**

Method:

1. Combine chicken, salsa, garlic, chili powder, chiles and salt and pepper.
2. Cover and cook on Low setting for 8 hours.
3. Transfer the chicken in a bowl and shred using two forks. Place it back in the slow cooker juices and serve in taco shells.
4. You can also top the shells with shredded cheese, sour cream or lime wedges, depending on your children's preferences.

Juicy Chicken Burgers

Serves: 8
Slow Cooker Size: 5- quart
Preparation time: 25 Minutes
Cooking Time: 4 Hours
Ingredients:

- 1 pound boneless, skinless chicken thighs cut in small pieces
- 1 pound boneless, skinless chicken breasts cut in small pieces
- 1 tbsp extra virgin olive oil
- Salt and pepper to taste
- 1 medium onion, diced
- 1 medium red bell pepper, seeded and diced
- 3 cloves garlic, roughly chopped
    - 1 can crushed tomatoes
- 3 tbsp Worcestershire sauce
- ¼ cup hot-pepper sauce
- 2 tbsp yellow mustard
- 1 tbsp molasses

- 8 buns
- Cucumber slices, tomato slices and lettuce leaves

Method:

1. Season the chicken with salt and pepper and cook on a large skillet in oil until golden brown on both sides, will take around 6 minutes.
2. Place the chicken in the slow cooker.
3. Add onions, bell pepper and garlic in the skillet and cook over medium heat for about 6 minutes or until the onions become translucent. Add ¼ cup of water and cook for another five minutes. Scrape the brown bits off from sides and season with salt and pepper.
4. Add this mixture to the slow cooker and top with the rest of the ingredients, except the buns.
5. Cover and cook on High setting for 4 hours.
6. Take out the chicken, shred using forks and mix it with the sauce again.

7. Serve on buns.

Cheesy Chicken and Broccoli

Serves: 4

Slow Cooker Size: 5- quart

Preparation time: 10 Minutes

Cooking Time: 7 Hours 20 Minutes

Ingredients:

- 4 boneless, skinless chicken breasts
- 1 ½ cup chicken broth
- 1 can cream of cheddar soup
- 1 can cream of chicken soup
- ¾ cup sour cream
- 3 tsp garlic powder
- 6 cups broccoli florets, cooked
- 2 cup cooked rice

Method:

1. Add chicken broth, cream of cheddar, cream of chicken, garlic powder and salt to the slow cooker and mix well. Add the chicken on the top.
2. Cover and cook on Low setting for 7 hours.

3. Transfer the chicken in a large bowl and shred using two forks.
4. Add the cooked broccoli and sour cream and cook for another 20 minutes on Low setting.
5. Serve with rice.

Juicy Chicken Breasts

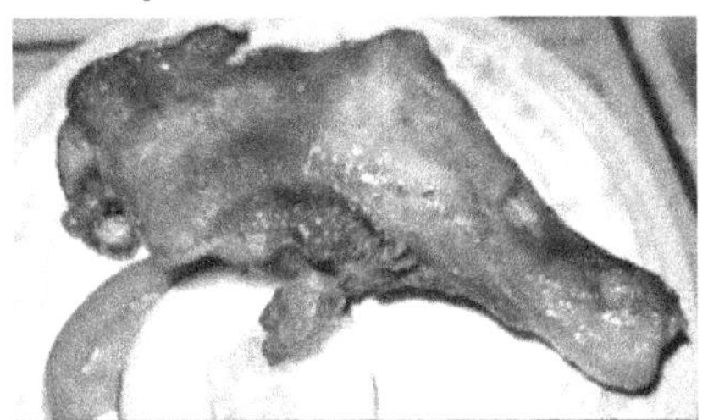

Serves: 4

Slow Cooker Size: 5- quart

Preparation time: 15 Minutes

Cooking Time: 4 Hours

Ingredients:

- 4 bone-in, skin on chicken breasts
- 2 tsp paprika
- 2 tbsp all purpose steak seasoning

Method:

1. Lay the bottom of the slow cooker with 5 foil balls.
2. Season the chicken breasts with paprika and steak seasoning.
3. Lay the chicken breasts on top of the foil in the slow cooker and cook on High setting for 4 hours.

4. Transfer the chicken on the serving dish
   and brush it with the juices from the
   slow cooker.

Chicken Teriyaki

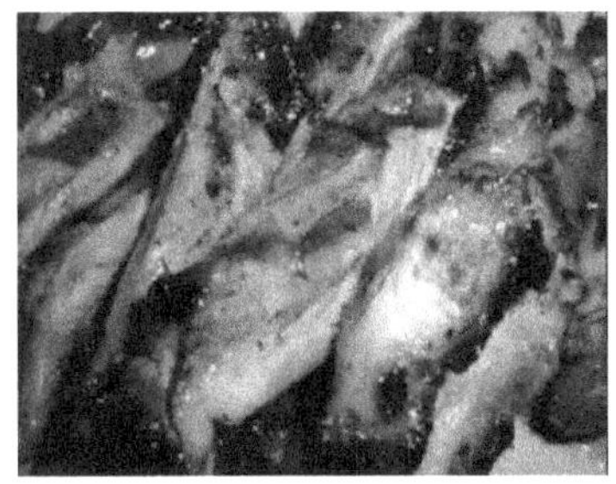

Serves: 4

Slow Cooker Size: 5- quart

Preparation time: 15 Minutes

Cooking Time: 7 Hours

Ingredients:

- 6 boneless chicken thighs
- 2 tbsp grated ginger
- 2 tbsp brown sugar
- ½ cup low sodium soy sauce
- 2 garlic cloves, minced

Method:

1. Add the chicken in the slow cooker along with the rest of the ingredients.

2. Cover and cook on High for one
   hour and then reduce the heat and
   cook on Low setting for 6 hours.
3. Serve on a bed of cooked rice or shred
   it and make sandwiches.

Chicken Meat Balls

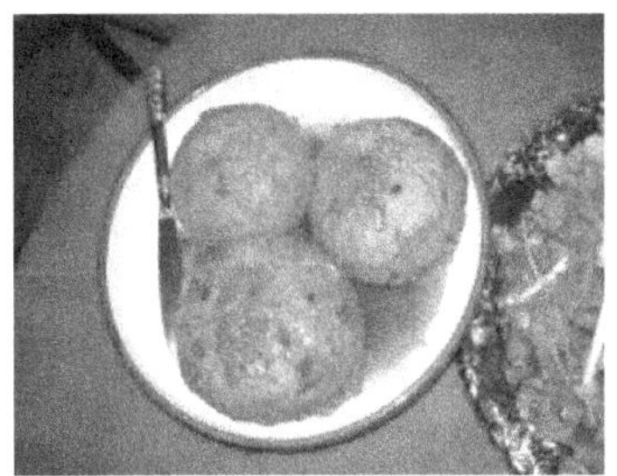

Serves: 6
Slow Cooker Size: 6- 7- quart
Preparation time: 25 Minutes
Cooking Time: 7-8 Hours
Ingredients:

For Marinara

- 2 tbsp extra virgin olive oil
- Pinch red pepper flakes
- 1 medium onion, finely chopped
- 1 tsp dried basil
- Two cans crushed tomatoes
- Salt and pepper to taste
- ½ cup finely chopped Italian parsley

For Chicken Meatballs

1. 2 pounds chicken

2. ¼ cup milk

3. 1 large egg, beaten

4. 1 cup bread crumbs

5. 2 tbsp Italian parsley

6. ½ cup grated Parmesan cheese

7. ½ cup finely chopped onion

8. Salt to taste

9. 1 clove garlic, minced

Method:

1. Heat oil in a small pan and sauté onion, garlic, basil and pepper flakes, around 5 minutes.

2. Transfer the onion mixture to the slow cooker and add salt, pepper, tomatoes and parsley on top. Mix well.

3. Cover and cook for 3 hours on Low setting.

4. Meanwhile, add the bread crumbs and milk in a large mixing bowl and mix. Add the rest of the ingredients and blend well.

5. Form 2-inch balls from the mixture. Transfer the meatballs in the slow

cooker and gently spoon some of the sauce over them.

6. Cover and cook for an additional 3 hours, or until the meatballs are fully cooked.

Smokey Chicken

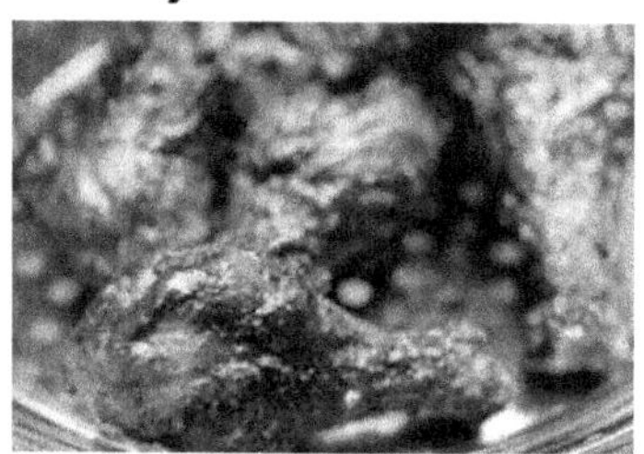

Serves: 5
Slow Cooker Size: 4- quart
Preparation time: 15 Minutes
Cooking Time: 7 Hours
Ingredients:

- 3 pounds skinned chicken pieces, including breast halves and thighs
- Salt and pepper to taste
- 1 cup chicken broth
- ½ cup snipped dried apricots
- 1 tbsp quick cooking tapioca, finely ground
- 1 tbsp adobo sauce
- 2 canned chipotle chile peppers in adobo sauce, chopped
- 111/2 cup raspberry jam

Method:

1. Season the chicken pieces with salt and pepper and place them in the slow cooker.
2. Stir raspberry jam, chipotle sauce, broth, adobo sauce and tapioca in a small bowl and pour over the chicken pieces.
3. Cover and cook on Low setting for 7 hours.

Puttanesca Chicken

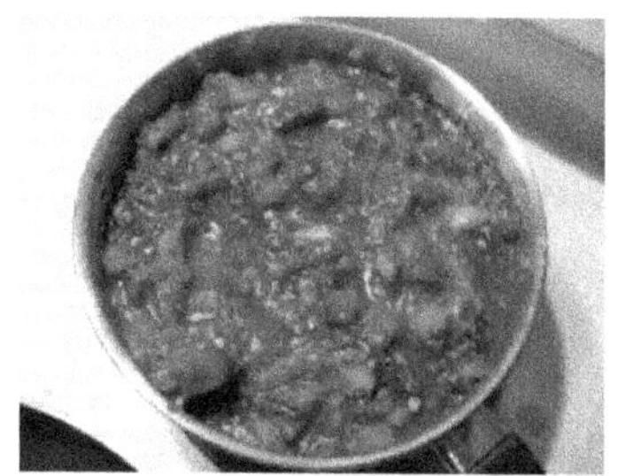

Serves: 6

Slow Cooker Size: 4- quart

Preparation time: 20 Minutes

Cooking Time: 7 Hours

Ingredients:

- 3 pounds skinless chicken pieces including drumsticks, thighs and breast halves
- 26 ounce jar pasta sauce with olives
- Salt and pepper to taste
- 3 cups cooked orzo pasta
- 2 tsp finely shredded lemon peel
- 2 tbsp drained capers

Method:

1. Season the chicken pieces with salt and pepper and place them in the slow cooker.
2. Mix capers, lemon peel and pasta sauce in a bowl and pour it over the chicken pieces.
3. Cover and cook on Low setting for 7 hours.
4. Serve the chicken over cooked orzo.

Conclusion

There you go! Scrumptiously divine chicken slow-cooker recipes to make each day, night, and special occasion feast a memorable one. Now you can easily throw away your Crock-pot carton, because from now on, your slow cooker will not need to be boxed ever again!

The greatest thing about slow cooker recipes are that they fit in well with a fast paced lives making it the perfect solution for working individuals and parents to easily prepare delectable meals. Simply prepare the ingredients in less than 15 minutes in the morning and come home to steaming hot and deliciously desirable meals in the evening.

Time to get inventive and start cooking!